SAVE
EVERY LIFE
YOU CAN

SAVE
EVERY LIFE
YOU CAN

A reflection on leadership and saving lives during the COVID-19 pandemic

RICHARD A. STONE M.D.

MAJOR GENERAL RETIRED, US ARMY
FORMER EXECUTIVE IN CHARGE/ACTING UNDER SECRETARY FOR HEALTH,
DEPARTMENT OF VETERANS AFFAIRS

MILL CITY PRESS

Mill City Press, Inc.
2301 Lucien Way #415
Maitland, FL 32751
407.339.4217
www.millcitypress.net

Library of Congress Control Number: 2022915876

Paperback ISBN-13: 978-1-6628-5342-5
Ebook ISBN-13: 978-1-6628-5343-2

To Jennifer, Rebecca, and Daniel
and to the memory of my father

Acknowledgments

LIKE ALL WORTHY PROJECTS, this book was envisioned and completed as a team. The author owes great debt to the team of Jon Jensen, Rosemary Williams, Brian Hawthorne, and Kate Shepard. These long-time colleagues and friends not only encouraged the development of the book but also contributed to its factual accuracy and coherent flow. They each believed in the validity of memorializing the events surrounding the COVID-19 pandemic even as the emotion of the losses from this horrific disease remained around us. I want to acknowledge and thank each of them for their extraordinary talent and belief in my ability to memorialize and reflect on the events and decisions we made.

Acknowledgment must also go to my wife Jenni, who has supported and believed in me for every moment we have been together.

Table of Contents

Introduction

THIS MANUSCRIPT WAS CREATED during the first half of calendar year 2022. As of June 2022, it has now been thirty-one months since the Veterans Health Administration (VHA) began its early response to the COVID-19 pandemic in December 2019. VHA has, as of June 2022, diagnosed and treated more than 684,030 cases of Veterans infected with the COVID-19 virus. More than 86,000 of those Veterans have been admitted to VHA hospitals for care. Tragically, VHA has also experienced the death of 22,262 of those Veterans infected, and 257 of VHA's own employees have been lost to COVID-19.[1] I served as the Veterans Health Administration executive in charge and then as the acting under secretary for health during much of this period. Under both titles and performing the duties of the under secretary for health from July 16, 2018, to July 16, 2021, I was responsible for ensuring the success of the nation's largest integrated health system through the pandemic.

I was further responsible and empowered to ensure the VHA could serve effectively as the "backstop" to overwhelmed civilian and Indian Health Service hospitals and nursing homes caring for COVID-19-infected patients across the nation. Beginning in December 2019, and as we progressed through the peaks and valleys of the pandemic, the VHA attempted to memorialize the events and challenges of this once-in-a-hundred-year public health emergency. It was anticipated that the chronology and challenges identified would be of use by future leaders and leadership teams. We prepared a chronology of events, documented actual, difficult lessons learned, and provided recommendations that those leaders who followed me at the VHA could continue to create and expand upon. As I read those documents now, I find that they are accurate and comprehensive, but they lack the personal stories that bring these once-in-a-hundred-year events to life, reminding both the citizen and historian that the battle against COVID-19 was fundamentally a human one despite the inhuman statistics that we are surrounded by.

In 1918, the Great Influenza overtook the world as the Western world fought WWI. Accurate death counts are unknown, but the Great influenza would be the deadliest plague in human history and would kill between 17 and 50 million people worldwide. That pandemic began in Haskell County, Kansas, and spread across the world, facilitated by the mobilization and congregation of soldiers in training locations of the United States Army in preparation for WWI. [2]

More than one hundred years later, the COVID-19 pandemic has infected 535 million and killed more than 6.3 million of the world's population as of June 2022. [3] Over a million of those killed were from the United States, where more than 87 million Americans have been infected. COVID-19 has been the greatest loss of human life from a single episodic disease in over one hundred years. [4]

Abraham Lincoln, prior to assuming the presidency in the turbulence of 1861, gave a series of lectures entitled "Lectures on Discoveries and Inventions" in 1858 and continuing into 1859. Diana Schaub, in her book, *His Greatest Speeches: How Lincoln Moved the Nation*, reminds us that Lincoln called writing "the great invention of the world"; it enables us "to converse with the dead, the absent, and the unborn, at all distances of time and space." [5]

I respectfully submit to the reader the following stories and leadership lessons of what it was like and what we experienced as we led America's largest health system, the Veterans Health Administration at the Department of Veterans Affairs, through the first eighteen months of this tragic pandemic. This is provided by the author in a sincere effort to offer a voice to those we have lost, who were not present, and who will follow us in future generations of leadership. There is no doubt that leadership challenges just as complex as those we faced will occur at some point in the future.

The first death of an American Veteran from COVID-19 occurred on March 4, 2020. Over the next twenty-eight months, there had been more than 22,000 Veteran deaths, of which 257 were VA's own employees. [6] The VHA, as I memorialize these events, has completed 196 state governor, tribal leader, and other federal government-requested "fourth missions," where they were called upon to support individual states' overwhelmed commercial health care systems. This support has occurred across forty-eight of the nation's fifty states, Puerto Rico, American Samoa, Guam, and the US Virgin Islands. These missions have deployed almost six thousand VHA employees into commercial, Indian Health Service, and Navajo Nation acute care hospitals, nursing homes, and other VHA facilities that needed the support of the extraordinary employees of the VHA.

These statistics, while impressive, seem incredibly sterile and do not tell the story of the dedicated employees of the VHA who responded to this public health emergency even at risk of their own lives, for it makes this pandemic seem ubiquitous or consistent when, in reality, it was not one public health emergency but hundreds, even thousands, that occurred differently in every state, city, community, and hospital, each affecting individual people and their families in unique ways. Similarly, the statistics do not tell the incredible personal story of a leader and leadership team working tirelessly to ensure the four missions of the Veterans Health Administration remained successful through the initial eighteen months of the COVID-19 pandemic.

As will be explained in considerable detail in subsequent chapters, the VHA provides care to almost ten million of the nation's Veterans as the VHA's "first" mission. The second and third missions of the VHA are education and research. The fourth and least understood of the VHA's missions is to be the "backstop" or safety net for American health care systems when flood, fire, earthquake, hurricane, or pandemic should overwhelm a region's commercial or government health delivery system, such as the Indian Health Service (IHS).

It is my sincere hope that a future leader will find within these pages support and a steady hand with which to guide their organization, no matter the size, along what I would describe as the "unpaved roads" of a challenge that was so unique that it hasn't occurred for more than one hundred years. In these events, there are no "usual" or well-developed processes, and leaders must improvise as the weaknesses of their delivery systems are revealed under the pressure of rapidly evolving current events.

A leader's success is often dependent upon their ability to provide agile decisions and engage their teams effectively in their response to the challenges they face, and it is my hope that these personal and sometimes very emotional stories from one leader's experience in the COVID-19 pandemic will help future leaders to successfully lead their organizations through what inevitably will be unforeseen and significant challenges to their ultimate success.

I have been called many things in my life, but at my core, I am a physician, serving for more than forty-five years in a profession and a calling that is fundamentally grounded in the relationship between a patient and the team caring for them. Early in my career, I focused entirely on the patient in front of me, then the patients on my ward, later across a facility, and so on. At each juncture of my career, I have noted that acts of kindness, compassion, and talent make all the difference in preserving health and society with the most precious and immeasurable gift: life.

It is my fervent hope that this document will contribute in some measure to future leaders' ability to face those challenges and *save every life they can.*

—Dr. Richard Stone

Prologue

I HAVE BEEN A STUDENT of leadership for what seems like my entire lifetime.

When I was fifteen years old, I had my first paid job as a stock handler at a large grocery chain. I encountered a leader in that job who was what one might call toxic. I couldn't understand the daily yelling by this manager at or toward employees, and attempts to defend my own actions were met with his vitriol.

Dinner in my house when I was a teenager was a sacred, uninterruptable, and often unappreciated (by my brother and me) ritual where Dad, sitting at the head of the table, engaged each of us on the events and challenges in our daily lives and solicited our opinions on world and local events. He encouraged honest discussion and would probe until truth was evident.

It came to pass that I decided that dinner would be the best time for me to announce that I was quitting my job because of this leader. I engaged my dad as soon as dinner began and explained my profound emotional discomfort with this leader. Dad paused a few moments, then smiled and said he understood my concern, but he could not support my intent to resign. He went on to discuss that over my entire working life, I would encounter leaders of different styles and types. He explained that all leaders were not like the one my fellow employees and I were struggling with. He further explained that each leader or manager gave a subordinate employee a gift. That gift was demonstrating that individual leader's model of leadership behavior. He noted that each of those encounters would add to my own style of leadership and demonstrate those traits that I would eventually want to emulate or reject. He finished our discussion with, "Aren't you lucky to encounter a leader like this so early in your employment career?" Somehow, I didn't feel lucky.

A month later, the toxic leader was replaced after a visit from the regional manager by an extraordinary, experienced, successful, and kind store manager that became a personal mentor and friend for more than thirty years of my life. When I related this change in managers and tone of my employment at a subsequent dinner, Dad again smiled and pointedly related that if I had resigned, I would have been denied the opportunity to see what extraordinary stabilizing individual leadership could deliver to a team.

Over the many decades that have followed, I have observed and worked for leaders that I was drawn to follow and those whose enduring lessons I sought not to mimic. They all molded me into the leader of the Veterans Health Administration that eventually faced the COVID-19 pandemic leading America's largest health care delivery system.

All my decisions during this unprecedented human tragedy were predicated upon the experiences I had assimilated in observing leadership over my lifetime. I ask the reader to spend time with the lessons of these stories, as they helped shape the leader that engaged this invisible, deadly, and massively destructive enemy.

I believe that leaders can be trained, formed, and developed. My service in the US Army allowed me to personally observe the development of competent young leaders who could be prepared, in just a few years, to lead the greatest soldiers on earth as non-commissioned officers. Certainly, the development of tactical and strategic vision formulates uniquely in individual leaders, but for each of us as leaders, the most important gift to our development is our experiences.

The gift my dad provided during that evening dinner conversation in my fifteenth year of life was to accept those lessons for what they are and what they could mold me to become. In order to understand my decisions decades later in facing the pandemic, I provide the reader with some of those extraordinary experiences in the following pages.

CHAPTER ONE

Bagram Airfield, Parwan Province, Afghanistan

MAY 2003

THE WHEELS OF THE giant Air Force cargo plane struck the runway with a jarring thud, awakening all of us. The back of an Air Force C-17 is a completely open space within a massive fuselage that can be configured for any mission need. It can be an airborne personnel transport, mail delivery aircraft, general-purpose heavy delivery transport aircraft, or even an intensive care unit. It can move mail, personnel, or trucks into the war and, in a few hours, be transformed into an advanced ICU taking grievously wounded service members away from the war to a place providing more complex care, accompanied by amazingly well-qualified and experienced Air Force medical personnel specially trained in critical care air transport and the nuances of providing care within a high-altitude pressurized space. This team's mission that day was to deliver a replacement Army combat hospital from Milwaukee, Wisconsin, to Bagram Airfield, Afghanistan. The plane was configured with web seats in a line down each side of the plane's fuselage. Our pallets of medical equipment and personal belongings were shrink-wrapped, strapped, and locked into the floors at the rear of the aircraft. Forward of the equipment was open space, and embedded in the front of the aircraft was crew areas and a couple of restrooms. The pilots climbed stairs in this area up to the cockpit controls, which were walled off from those of us in the back cargo space. The rear of the aircraft at flying altitude was very cold, with most heat coming from the front of the fuselage. We could see our breath as we exhaled, and most of us were wrapped in blankets. It was May 2003. I was commanding the United States Army Reserve's 452nd Combat Hospital, having assumed command just before September 11, 2001, and had hand-selected the 148 medical and support soldiers that were now preparing to land in Afghanistan. Our mission was to replace another Army hospital unit and operate as the primary delivery site for complex trauma care throughout the war in Afghanistan.

As soon as the plane landed and slowed to a taxi speed, the loadmaster opened the giant rear ramp as large as a two-lane highway and exposed the entire back of the plane to the outside. The ramp seemed like a roadway tunnel opening with massive hydraulics so that the far edge was just above the ground and the entire rear of the aircraft was open. There were few windows along the sides of the fuselage of this plane, and the bright, warm noontime sun surprised all of us. The air was hot, and the dust was everywhere inside the plane as soon as the ramp opened. The plane turned, and for the first time, I saw what would become my home for the next year.

Bagram Airfield was a massive single runway built in the 1950s and expanded by the Russians during their occupation of Afghanistan from December 1979 until February 1989. It was in the high desert (about 5000 feet above sea level or approximately the same elevation as the city of Denver), and it was surrounded by the Hindu Kush mountains. The more than a mile of runway was lined on one entire side by low one- and two-story buildings and what seemed like an entire city of tents and buildings that extended for nearly a mile and ran the entire length of the runway. On the opposite side was an extensive rock-filled desert, flat areas of sand and rocks and piles of debris of war to include multiple types of Russian military airplanes that had been abandoned when the Soviet military fled the onslaught of the Mujahedeen, who, under the leadership of their brilliant commander, Ahmad Shah Massoud, had ridden on horseback through the minefields to surprise and overwhelm the Russians. The Russians had attempted to protect the massive perimeter with a huge number of land mines deployed randomly in order to protect from just such an assault. This attack in 1982 was followed by seven more years of losses by the Russians in a failed effort to make Afghanistan a satellite of the Soviet Union. The Russians abandoned this war in 1989.

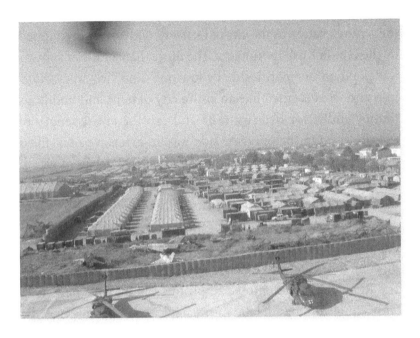

P1: Bagram Airfield during a helicopter landing. Note minefield with debris of war in front of the US Army Hospital ER entrance.

—

As I stepped off the back ramp of the C-17, I was ushered into a line of soldiers waiting to register our arrival on the giant air base. The Air Force was the same as the Army, inefficient in this type of personnel service and able to create an endless line almost instantaneously. It always amazed me that an organization that could operate such complex airborne platforms could falter on even the most basic of human resource-related processes. The Army was no better, and I suspect the Navy is about the same. Standing in line for almost everything in the Army is where I began saying how wonderful it was that the Army paid us the same, whether we were productive or not.

As I stood in this line, a tall, thin, bald, and suntanned colonel in an Army physical fitness uniform with a 9mm pistol shoulder holstered under his left arm grabbed my hand and shook it firmly. "Colonel Stone, I am Colonel Hector Henry, the medical task force commander. Welcome to Bagram. Get signed in, find your tent, and rest; you're tired, and there is lots to do. I'm going to go run." And with that, he turned and was gone. It was as he turned that I recognized that this man had the largest ears I had ever seen. I discovered later that the colonel was an avid runner who only ran when the days heat had reached its peak. A Vietnam War-era Veteran and trained urologic surgeon, he loved the Army and the Fort Bragg "Airborne" culture. He could not speak of his beloved Army and its soldiers without tearing up and his voice breaking, no matter if he was speaking to a single soldier or the entire task force. I would come to love him as "my brother from another mother." Our friendship would last until his death in 2013 from a rare blood cancer that Hector was convinced was caused by the airborne hazards and burn pits that we lived next to and inhaled smoke from for those many months.

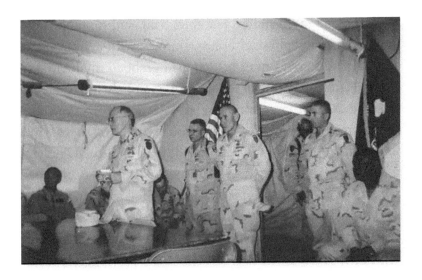

P2: COL Hector Henry standing behind then Army Surgeon General James Peake. Bagram Afghanistan, 2003. (Author to Colonel Henry's right)

—

I completed the sign-in process and was met by some of my advance party that had arrived the previous day. We walked from the airfield to the main street of this thriving military city encased in the secure perimeter. There were thousands of soldiers, airmen, Marines, and even a few Navy personnel walking everywhere. The main street was unpaved and dusty. Small rocks were everywhere to firm up the road and sidewalk. Makeshift sidewalks paralleled one side of the road. Bizarre civilian trucks decorated in bright paint and chains rumbled at five to ten miles per hour down the road. These "jingle trucks" were driven by Afghan and Pakistani drivers who hauled most of our supplies from ports in Pakistan. This, I was later informed, was dangerous work, and these drivers were frequently attacked by the enemy and local bandits for their cargo, often losing their lives or, at the very least, their vehicles and cargo. Even our fuel was obtained by these trucks, the sounds of their dangling chains warning of their approach. We could only obtain jet fuel through our supply lines, and most of our ground vehicles were diesel-powered. Our mechanics would mix the jet fuel with oil to allow the wheeled vehicles to run. I quickly gained extraordinary respect for our mechanics who seemed could adapt or fix anything.

Farther away from the road were lines of HESCO barriers and sandbags stacked eight to ten feet high. The HESCO was invented by a British coal miner turned entrepreneur. These containers were composed of chicken wire-like wire configurations and lined with potato sack-like material. They appeared like three dimensional rectangular containers that could be transported empty to a particular location, filled with rocks and dirt, and then stacked one upon the other to make barriers in any location. Their name is a portmanteau of the inventor's name and the word concertina.

As we walked, the leader of my advance team discussed the value of these barriers in reducing the danger of the then nearly daily rocket and mortar attacks that primarily came from the neighborhoods outside our perimeter in the adjacent city of Bagram. Bagram airfield had a single external gate that was intentionally tortuous and separated vehicles into discrete areas for robust inspection of each vehicle and its contents before the vehicle and its driver could enter the military base. Multiple explosives-detecting working dogs supported this continuous operation.

As we walked along the street, I could feel the sand blowing against my face from the ever-present wind. My escort laughed and said it was like an antiaging facial "peel" done daily by the wind to keep us looking young. A year later, I had replaced my eyeglasses three times because of the pitting on the lenses from the daily sand blasting. I would also develop a persistent cough from inhaling the airborne materials. That cough has now become permanent, and the debate over burn pits and airborne hazard is clear in my mind.

About a half mile down the road, on the tarmac side of the blast enclosures was the entrance to the combat hospital compound. It was marked by a giant red cross and a sign that gave the heat index and advice on what each heat category meant. My escort talked about how long it would take to truly acclimatize to the heat and elevation. I was advised running was prohibited for the first few days after arrival. The hospital was completely sandbagged from the ground up to about four feet, and the entrances formed an irregular maze to prevent an explosive blast wave from entering the care and personnel areas. Most of the hospital was covered with camouflage netting to reduce the heat in the tents underneath. Living quarters surrounded the hospital, also composed of tents. The hospital was composed of both tents and firm-sided shipping container-like metal boxes configured in a trademarked system called DEPMEDS (deployable medical systems) that the Army uses as standardized modular and deployable field hospitals. We had trained on this system for many years. Outside the emergency room entrance was a parking area that placed the vehicles up against a fence of barbed wire, beyond which were two abandoned Russian MiG-23 aircraft. These abandoned aircraft were painted with graffiti in mostly English and sat on uneven ground. The area of barbed wire fencing was marked with "Do not enter **MINES**–Explosion Hazard" every few feet. I was told it was too dangerous to sweep, identify, and remove the mines from this area because we would have to close and evacuate the hospital during the minesweeping process. The ICU and general medical nursing units were soft-sided rectangular tents covered in ever-present dust, and the ORs, lab, and pharmacy were sand-colored metal-walled boxes that looked like shipping containers when transported but then were opened on the side walls to expand to triple their width. All of this tentage and containers were connected by passage-ways to completely climate control the hospital and attempt to reduce the ever-present sand from entering the facility. As I approached the living quarters placed around the perimeter, I noted that some had heaters to protect from the high desert cold nights. Temperatures in the winter in the high desert could fall to below zero. As the hospital commander, I was offered a small 500-square-foot mud-walled house that I was told was heated and air-conditioned. It was close to the medical task force headquarters tent. I refused the offer. I wanted to live in the same quarters as my soldiers. My escort shrugged, and I was quickly assigned to a six-person tent that had been placed along the taxiway where the US Air Force A-10 close air support aircraft were positioned. These fairly slow-moving but highly lethal aircraft ran constantly to provide rapid protection to the base perimeter and the supported theater of operations. They are very loud and part of the reason I now wear hearing aids.

I was assigned to a tent with a number of other physicians, nurses, and my deputy commander, another physician by the name of Rick Haile. Rick would become an extraordinary partner in all phases of combat operations, and when I was moved to become medical Task Force commander replacing Colonel Henry when he redeployed home to Ft. Bragg, Rick became commander of the combat hospital. The personnel of the hospital unit we were replacing had vacated the living areas and moved off the compound. They would come back to the compound as we would execute what was called a left seat right seat orientation for my soldiers over several shifts to ensure no patient or staff was placed at risk before or after the official hand-off of responsibilities.

I was given the following instructions by my new compound (company) commander: sleep as low to the ground as you can as mortars come nearly every night. "Let's not lose you to a lucky shot, sir." I decided I would sleep in a low cot in my portion of the tent. My personal gear was delivered from the pallets, and I established my "home" by connecting pictures of my wife and children on tent lines hanging from the wall with clothes pins I had brought from home.

I laid down for just a moment and fell asleep immediately for what seemed like a few minutes but was for the rest of the afternoon. I was awakened by what seemed like a tornado warning siren. I grew up in the Midwest in areas prone to tornados and knew that the siren meant "seek cover." I had no idea where to go, and no one else was in the tent. I left the tent through the door tent flaps to the outside. It was pitch black in every direction. I was immediately lost.

I don't remember ever experiencing such complete darkness. There was nothing to orient to except the noise of generators everywhere. The inside of the tent had light bulbs hanging from the ceiling, and although dim, it was easy to see. I stumbled as my night vision was not well practiced. I found the flaps and ropes to the tent entrance behind me. I reentered the tent and was searching for my red lens flashlight when the first explosion occurred. I estimated that it was at least a half mile away. Over the next few months, I would become an expert in this blast distance estimation. But even so, the blast pressure wave rippled the loose flaps of the tent, and I could feel the blast pressure wave against my chest. I stopped for just a second to see if there were going to be more. It seemed like at least a minute between the warning and the impact. I resolved to figure out where the bunker my escort had casually discussed was actually located and how long it would take me to get there. I further resolved to find my way to the health operations center (medical task force command tent) to check on casualties.

Twenty minutes later, I found my way to the ER entrance. No casualties were being treated, no one had left their post to go to the bunker, and no one seemed overly phased by the attack. The universal response was, "The bad guys are not very good shots." I smiled, thanked them for their bravery, and found the health operations center. My operations officer, an energetic, bright major by the name of Bill Klemp, and a highly experienced NCO Miguel Moyeno (master sergeant) responded to my presence by admonishing me that I should be in the bunker. *I was too valuable to lose.* It seemed to me that that was an extraordinarily inane statement. They both had the skills to engage in and manage our response to this attack and our response to potential casualties. Their expertise was the centerpiece of managing our response. I was just the guy who had been lost in the dark. I vowed at that point that during any attack or operational challenge, I would be right next to them as quickly as possible. They were the subject matter experts, and the best thing I could do to make my decisions better was to defer to their expertise. This was one of my first lessons of combat.

The major and master sergeant then briefed me on the location of the mortar impact. I was lucky to have them both with me. They were experienced, calm, and professional. The all-clear siren sounded as they briefed me; no damage and no casualties. The origin of the mortar was the town next to us. The enemy, Major Klemp briefed, entered the walled compounds of local families' homes in the city next to our perimeter, fired the mortars or rockets, and then left immediately. This, the enemy believed, would reduce the chance our artillery would respond and risk civilian casualties.

How did we know all this so quickly to even activate the warning system? The answer was that we possessed what was called "ground effect radar," which picked up the projectile as soon as it was fired, plotted the trajectory, and identified the grid coordinates of the origin point. It was believed that information was fed to our artillery batteries, and we could respond in less than a minute. We never did. The risk of our response to civilians was so significant that our leadership had decided it wasn't worth the risk. I was also informed that all these decisions were made in the Combined Joint Task Force (CJTF) 180 Operations Center about a half mile down the road near where we had signed in. I was also told that we had a "office" there, and we were at the present time working that "office" remotely from where I was standing. I vowed to go there the next day to ensure I completely understood this capability. I returned to my tent but walked through the hospital. The hospital was filled with Americans and Afghans injured in the war. All of the US medical personnel were busy, engaged, kind, and pleasant. I left the back of one of the ICU units and was met again by the absolutely oppressive blackness of the night. I had my flashlight in hand and used the red-lensed light to find my way back to my tent. I would have to get better at this.

The next morning, Colonel Henry walked me to the CJTF 180 operations center that I was informed of the previous night. It looked like an indoor tennis bubble or golf dome. It was higher on one end than the other and appeared to me to be an inflatable dome structure made of thick plastic material. The roar of generators surrounded the outside. We traversed the maze of sandbags to enter, featuring a more robust maze than the hospital compound entrance. We registered with the guards and entered behind what appeared to be a set of bleachers inside the dome. We walked around the side, and as the front of the bleachers came into view, I visually oriented to multiple massive TV screens and maps projected on screens located at the low end of the dome. The bleachers faced these screens, and each level of the bleachers was filled with simple flat desks. Each desk was equipped with a computer screen and keyboard, and seated at each desk were personnel working the activities of managing this war. Each desk had a placard hanging from the front edge of the desk identifying the expertise of those working in that location. Around the sides of the dome were passageways leading to long well-lit tents with additional desks. Each was marked with identifying signs along the tent wall. Colonel Henry directed me to the seat beside him at a desk marked for the medical Task Force commander. Colonel Henry put on headphones with a microphone and handed me a pair of headphones, and the morning briefing began.

In the ensuing thirty minutes the commander of all US forces in Afghanistan would see and hear from every leader across Afghanistan and our supporting forces in Uzbekistan. He sat at the lowest level of the bleachers in the center of the front row facing the screens. He listened and made decisions immediately. No one across the entire field of operations had to guess what he was thinking or his intended direction. There was complete transparency of decision-making and how each of us needed to orient ourselves to the challenges that faced us. Nothing was left out. When Colonel Henry briefed, it was concise and focused. It was also delivered with a profound North Carolinian accent.

"General, there are no bed, personnel, or material shortages in the medical Task Force. Blood supply is adequate for tonight's operations. The replacement hospital personnel and their command has arrived. Colonel Stone is with me observing this briefing." It took less than thirty seconds. The commander knew everything he needed to know. It was the same for everything from air operations, brigade combat units, logistics, etcetera, and even the State Department liaison briefed. It was all in the same manner, concise and focused on the mission. The commanding general (CG) asked an occasional question and reserved his direction to the end unless corrections were needed.

There was a huge learning opportunity here. Every day my thought would become, *What information do I need to give to the CG, and what direction or support do I need from anyone else on the team?* I was stunned at the efficiency and professionalism I would learn from this group of leaders every single day. Lessons in leadership can occur in any venue as long as you are listening, even in what appeared to be a converted golf dome in the middle of Afghanistan.

CHAPTER TWO

The Safety Patrol

AUGUST 1962 – JUNE 1963

OVER MY LIFETIME, I have learned many lessons in leadership. Some started very early.

I was in fifth grade, at age eleven, and we were living in Mt. Clemens, Michigan. This was a town of about 35,000 people at that time that was located about thirty miles northeast of the city of Detroit. Mt. Clemens is a community with a long and storied history. It was the center of mineral bath therapy for arthritis patients during the Prohibition era drawing worldwide visitors for warm mineral bath treatments for crippling diseases, such as arthritis and post-polio limb contractures. It also was the centerpiece of illegal liquor manufacturing during Prohibition, resulting in a profoundly wealthy community. By the 1950s and early 1960s, when I was in elementary school, most of that wealth had dissipated, and Mt. Clemens was a quiet business community that had been designated as the center of the county government, drawing a large number of legal professionals that supported the town's economy.

It was here that I recall my first exposure to serving in a leadership position. I had decided that I would apply to become the leader (captain) of the Lincoln Elementary School Safety Patrol. I was intrigued with the authority that each of the Safety Patrol members displayed, and my mother, I had witnessed, was constantly lecturing my older brother on community service. I thought this was a chance to avoid the ire thus far Mom had directed solely at him.

—

The position of leader of the Safety Patrol was an elected position, chosen by the entire student body of the Lincoln Elementary School. The school was, even then, an ancient multi-storied brick building with classrooms on each floor and in the basement. Atop the roof was a cupola of wood painted white and flying the American flag from its highest point. In the basement were designated community "fallout" shelters as located a few miles to our east was an Air Force base that was home to the Strategic Air Command. This base housed some number of B-52 aircraft capable of delivering nuclear bombs around the world. Attached to the outside of the school entrances were placed large yellow and black "fallout shelter" signage, and we as elementary school students practiced hiding under our desks, covering our heads, and then quickly congregating all the students and staff in the basement because we knew that the nearby military base was a primary Russian target. We had just experienced the Cuban missile crisis of 1961, and we were all confident that we had the best place in the city to survive a nuclear attack.

I walked to and from school each day. We lived only three blocks away from the school and lived on the same street as the Sisters of Charity St Joseph Hospital, an ancient sanitarium-type building that arose as a tuberculosis sanitarium and delivered mineral baths as it sat atop a mineral water well. When the well water was pumped, it left an acrid stench across the neighborhood that all of us learned to ignore. While walking to school, there was one significant road to cross. That road had a traffic light and was one lane each way. The student crossing point was staffed by fifth and sixth-grade Safety Patrol "officers"; no parents, no police, and no educational staff from the school, just students wearing a white belt that extended over the shoulder and around the waist and who had been trained by the student leadership of the Safety Patrol.

Captain of the Safety Patrol was the job I was running for, and there were three of us hoping to be elected to this position. We were all friends and played on the same Little League baseball team. When I found out that my two friends were running, I remained confident I would win the election. I had no platform to run on, just a desire to serve, enabled by my mom and my impression that the Safety Patrol officers were respected members of the school community. The day before the election, the three of us candidates walked from classroom to classroom in the four-story building, each of us providing a short two-minute speech about why we should be considered for this position and deserved the students vote. We spoke to the entire electorate. This was part of a civics class for the entire school on the responsibilities of voting, citizenship, and how elections were conducted. The next morning, the election was held in each class. I couldn't sleep the night after the speeches. I was excited to win, although I thought my speech was clearly the least impressive of the three candidates. When the votes were counted, I came in third place. First place became captain, second became first lieutenant, and third place (me) became the second lieutenant. I have often wondered if there had ever been a second lieutenant before me, as it felt somewhat like a consolation prize, but I was proud of my new rank.

My responsibilities as second lieutenant included riding my bike from corner to corner and intersection to intersection around the school, assuring that each crossing guard was meeting performance standards and providing spot correction to each of them if any problems were discovered.

—

The lessons of this work were enormous and have stayed with me all these years.

What does management do when someone doesn't show up for work? Fortunately, this was a rare occurrence because everyone was so proud to serve and wear the belt. (After all, we were the community fallout shelter.) The simple answer was that the other lieutenant and I were the backup employees. What has stayed with me, however, is that employees who are connected to the mission will perform well beyond your expectations, even when illness or other distractions might take them away.

How does management assure common performance standards? There is no substitute for firsthand observation of an employee's performance. Deviation from the standard can be easily corrected with immediate spot corrections. This must be done with gentleness and compassion. Always assume individuals want to do the right thing and that errors should be viewed as exactly that, errors of execution, not errors of intent. Accept the fact that "to err is human" and build it into managing teams. This was another message from my mom, who was not quite as tolerant as I remember I was in the performance of my duties, nor were her responses to my errors as gentle.

An example of Mom's response to "unintended errors" follows. One of the responsibilities my brother and I assumed while growing up was to clean our room. My brother and I shared a finished attic in our small house before my parents divorced and we moved in with my grandparents. In executing my task of dusting, I, unfortunately, broke one of my older brother's model aircraft he had worked many weeks to complete. He was not pleased with my lack of care, and a physical altercation began between us. He never quite accepted the concept of "to err is human." Much later, I realized that immediate spot correction of my dusting ability could have avoided all of this. He was four years older, and the outcome of physical interaction was always predetermined. The outcome was never in my favor. My response was, therefore, to run, and in an effort to slow my brother in his pursuit of me, I launched a nearby shoe over my shoulder. My brother ducked, and the shoe sailed through the window glass at the end of the attic dormer. The shoe lodged itself in the outer plate of glass. This gained Mom's attention as glass went flying everywhere. Mom was not pleased, and the punishment included discipline directed to me for being careless and for throwing the shoe. Discipline was also directed to my brother (under protest) for ducking, as it was "only a tennis shoe" and wouldn't have hurt much if it hit him.

A leader must see all the work of the safety team stationed on corners with their own eyes. None of this work could be done sitting in an office. Leaders must lead by walking around (or riding their bike). The captain had a small desk outside the principal's office and, as directed by the principal, he stayed at that desk continuously from forty-five minutes before school began to one hour after school ended. The lieutenants were "on the road" continuously except for five minutes at the beginning and end of each day when we discussed any concerns the captain had about the work being performed. Quickly, we discovered his position was of no (or at least of little) value. Not because he was incompetent or ill-intentioned, but because he was so distant from the action of ensuring safety. He quickly lost the respect of those in the field doing work in the rain, snow, and cold of the Michigan school year.

I found the process of running for election demeaning and vowed I would never again run for public office. I have no idea why every "friend" discussed their vote with me. It seemed no one had voted for me. It taught an important lesson, however: popularity has little to do with the quality of a leader. Make the best out of any situation, even if you don't think it was where you should be. Get over it and do the best you can. Understanding the mission, enforcing standards fairly, and recognizing failure as uniquely human qualities were much more important than popularity to mission success.

Fairness created followership and earned the respect of those around you. Being willing to step in when employees needed help and removing employees when they could not do the mission had to be transparent and fair. Even a popular employee who could not perform endangered the mission, which was the safety of the student population. That employee must be mentored first, and if no improvement occurred, moving the employee to a more appropriate position was absolutely warranted.

All the above has stayed with me now almost sixty years later. It was an amazing opportunity for a lost election. I was fortunate to serve for both fifth and sixth grade until my family moved and changed school systems. The sense of loss in that move was overwhelming, and I have often wondered why. The move was predicated because my mom had remarried, and we had gone from living with my grandparents in a small 900-square-foot house with one bathroom serving five of us.

We were facing the possibility that we would become a family with a mom, dad, and my older brother with the arrival of a "dad." I had not experienced a normal family before. My biological father was an abusive alcoholic who my mom had divorced years earlier at a time when women did not often escape those situations. Her strength was enormous. Mom had told us that my brother and I were about to have our own bedrooms and our own beds for the first time. Life seemed like it was going to be much better. We were even promised a bathroom for the two of us.

My separation from the Safety Patrol team and the mission to ensure my fellow students' safety that I found myself so connected to, was the cause of the great sense of impending loss. I never went back after we moved out of the Mt. Clemens school district, but my feeling of abandoning my post and my responsibilities overwhelmed even what appeared to be enormously positive developments in our new family life. These feelings of abandonment would repeat themselves throughout my military and leadership career. I loved every job, no matter the challenge, and grieved leaving each one until I was able to connect to the next position and the people serving with me.

Over these many decades, I have had the opportunity to lead sports teams as a captain and then as a coach, served as a sergeant in the fire service, developed and led closely-held business partnerships, commanded soldiers in and out of combat, and finally, found myself leading America's largest health care system, The Veterans Health Administration through the initial eighteen months of the COVID-19 pandemic.

What follows is the extraordinary story of the difficult decisions we, as the Veterans Health Administration leadership team, and that I, individually, made during the COVID-19 pandemic. This includes both the success and failure that resulted from those decisions. For the reader looking for salacious stories, you will be sadly disappointed. There are those who served in leadership who were successful and those who were not. The stories that I will relate are told in a sincere effort to help all of you who aspire to or presently serve in leadership positions of any type. These stories are told to help you to traverse the challenges that you will ultimately face as you lead the members of your organization toward success at any level. These are ultimately the lessons we, as the leaders of VHA, learned in a once-in-a-hundred-year pandemic where an entire nation and nearly ten million Veterans depended upon us.

CHAPTER THREE

The Beginning

DECEMBER 2019 TO MARCH 2020

IN LATE DECEMBER 2019, the US government began to wind down operations for the Christmas holidays and New Year as usually occurs across the federal government beginning in mid-December. Congress departs Washington, DC, for their Christmas holiday, federal employees are looking forward to time with their families, and the city seems to take on a different tone. I was serving at this time as the executive in charge of the Veterans Health Administration (VHA). This essentially means I was performing the duties of the under secretary for health for the Veterans Health Administration. The under secretary is the "CEO" of America's largest health care system and the largest health delivery system in the US government. The under secretary for health is a presidentially nominated and senate confirmed political appointee. For the VHA, and other agencies, this can be a long and arduous process that includes seating a commission that interviews and recommends to the president three candidates that are endorsed and prioritized by the secretary of the VA, usually leading to one being nominated for the position. In the absence of a Senate-confirmed nominee, the government usually selects a senior government employee to serve until a political nominee is selected. I had served as the executive in charge of VHA since July 2018, reflecting the complexity of nominating and confirming a political leader to serve as the under secretary for this large and complex health system.

The VHA exists to provide lifetime health promotion and health care to all eligible veterans of uniformed federal service in the Army, Navy, Air Force, and Marine Corps. VHA is one of three subordinate agencies under the control of the cabinet secretary of the Department of Veterans Affairs (VA). The other two agencies of the VA are the Veterans Benefit Administration (VBA) and the National Cemetery Administration (NCA). The Department of Veterans Affairs exists as a sort of holding company providing oversight, strategic direction, and budget guidance to the three subordinate agencies, each led by under secretaries.

About half of America's nearly 19 million Veterans are enrolled in and depend on the VHA for their health care. [7] Although over 85 percent of American Veterans have other health insurance, usually provided by their employers, Veterans that are enrolled in VHA health care almost universally prefer to be cared for by a system and providers that are completely dedicated to their health and understand the unique health care needs resulting from military service. You wouldn't know it from the usual stories you see in the media about VHA, but Veterans are overwhelmingly satisfied with their care, and in recent surveys, about 89 percent of Veterans "trust" VHA and would recommend care in the VHA to their fellow Veterans. [8] (Author's note: Throughout the book, you will notice Veteran is capitalized. This is consistent with the writing style for VA, which is now habit, and I believe requires capitalization.)

VHA health care is delivered from 175 hospitals and about 1250 outpatient clinics dispersed across the nation, Puerto Rico, Virgin Islands, Guam, Saipan, American Samoa, and the Philippines. Wherever American Veterans are, the VHA either provides or buys care in the community to support them. The VHA purchases significant amounts of specialty care in areas where there is a shortage of specialists in order to assure access standards are met to support Veteran needs.

In addition, VHA provides world-class research on illnesses unique to or prevalent in the Veteran population, as well as combat-related injuries and illnesses. VHA operates advanced polytrauma rehabilitation centers, spinal cord care centers, and the world's most advanced blind rehabilitation system of care. In addition to care, since the end of WWII, VHA has developed academic affiliations that provide education to more than one hundred and twenty thousand physician residents in training, interns, and medical students in its facilities each day, making it the largest provider of medical education in the nation. Those who have argued for privatization and, therefore, dissolution of VHA fail to recognize that the entire American post-graduate medical education system would collapse without a robust and healthy VHA, not to mention dramatically reduced awareness of the unique medical and mental health challenges of those who have defended our nation's freedom. More on this topic later.

VHA's response to the pandemic is the focus of the pages that follow. We will attempt to tell the personal stories of how VHA successfully accomplished each of its four congressionally mandated missions through the first eighteen months of the pandemic. The VHA's fourth mission (emergency management) will be the focus of many of the lessons learned, but leadership lessons occurred as all four missions were challenged by the pandemic.

As mentioned in the introduction, the VHA provides care to 9 million Veterans of uniformed service as its first mission. The second and third mission of VHA is education and research, and the fourth mission is to be the backstop of America's regional health care systems in the event of a flood, earthquake, hurricane, or any other natural or manmade disaster that overwhelms the nation's civilian health care delivery systems.

The VHA website describes the fourth mission as follows:

> VA's fourth mission is to improve the nations preparedness for response to war, terrorism, national emergencies, and natural disasters by developing plans and taking action to ensure continued service to Veterans, as well as to support national, state and local emergency management, public health, safety and homeland security efforts.

This fourth mission has been in place for more than thirty years. It is part of Public Law 100–707 of federal law. The VA portion of the federal emergency medical response is triggered under the 1988 Stafford Disaster Relief and Emergency Assistance Act. [9]

Activation of the Stafford Act requires presidential declaration of an emergency and is usually further initiated by a state's governor asking the president of the United States for federal support when state or local assets are overwhelmed. [10]

Since 1988, the VHA has quietly provided regional support to communities after a hurricane, earthquake, or manmade event, contributing personnel and equipment and even mobile treatment units or ER beds. The capabilities of the VHA's Office of Emergency Management (OEM), responsible for executing this mission, have grown consistently over the more than three decades since the Stafford Act was passed by Congress to meet these needs.

Until COVID-19, all VHA "fourth mission" responses were limited to regional or even local emergencies. Each VHA mission was staffed with VHA employees who served as volunteers and entered as emergency responders after the tornado, hurricane, earthquake, or flood had passed. In essence, the entire response system had been designed to be agile and responsive but to deliver support *after* the danger had passed. This was always done with VHA employee volunteers, and those volunteers came from regions of the nation unaffected by the disaster. One of the best examples of this agile response occurred on June 12, 2016, when the VHA sent more than forty-five mental health providers to Orlando following the Pulse nightclub shooting when forty-nine people were killed and fifty-three wounded by a single shooter. We deployed within a few hours in support of local and federal law enforcement authorities who had requested that we assist during the process of reuniting and the identification of victims and their families. Other than the families and law enforcement personnel present, few Americans knew we were even there supporting the community following this horrific tragedy.

VHA employees from Louisiana also consistently volunteered for multiple fourth mission deployments following recovery from Hurricane Katrina in August 2005 that had devastated New Orleans, Louisiana. Universally, when meeting these volunteers during deployments, they each had a sense of giving back to communities that had supported their own families after the massive destruction of Katrina. They volunteered in an effort to say thank you for the support they, their families, and their community had received in 2005.

This is what the fourth mission was designed to be—temporary and local. Never had this VHA response capability been called upon to deploy nationwide, nor had we ever had to coordinate a simultaneous sustained emergency response. None of us had ever contemplated the need for a fifty-state and territory simultaneous response capability where every community was being affected.

There was one man who had contemplated just such a disaster, and he called me just before New Year's Eve 2019 and told me something I hope that I never hear again. I, like most government employees, was at home outside of Washington, DC, preparing for a prolonged quiet holiday with family and friends when my personal cell phone rang.

Paul Kim, MD, served as the executive director of the VHA Office of Emergency Management. He was a trained psychologist from Fordham University and received his MD from the Universidad de Ciudad Juarez, Mexico. Paul is extensively experienced and possesses certifications in federal emergency management, hazardous material response, medical management of weapons of mass destruction casualties, incident management, and emergency preparedness. In short, it's his job to plan for the worst while the rest of us hope for the best. Paul's position as executive director of the Office of Emergency Management (OEM) reported directly to Renee Oshinski, the chief of health care operations for VHA.

Paul had extensive experience at the New York City World Trade Center ground zero emergency response after the

September 11, 2001, terrorist attack, where he served on-site for the state of New York for over thirty days. He is an unflappable professional whom I came to respect and admire immensely. When Paul called me, he was leading a staff of one hundred subject matter experts in emergency response stationed in Martinsburg, West Virginia.

As I answered the phone, I fully expected a "happy holidays" message. Paul, however, was apologetic for disturbing my holidays, then quickly turned to a very direct message. Paul related the emerging knowledge of a new virus that was affecting Wuhan, China, and he warned that the possibility of spread to humans and subsequent human-to-human transmission that could lead to worldwide spread was imminent. He related a December 12th report from the Wuhan Municipal Health Commission that documented twenty-seven cases of pneumonia in customers who had purchased poultry, snakes, bats, and other foods at the Huanan Seafood Wholesale Market. He told me that we did not yet know the lethality of the virus, and he recommended that the VHA immediately begin preparations. We talked about the worldwide response to the 2013–2016 Ebola virus in West Africa. Like most serving in military medicine at that time, I was intimately familiar with the worldwide and US response as the world attempted to contain that threat. In the United States, we had seen only eleven patients with Ebola. Paul reminded me that Ebola had killed more than 11,000 people, primarily in West Africa. We both agreed that this was a terrible cost of lives. We agreed that preparations to ensure VHA readiness should begin immediately. Paul mobilized his team to action, and I informed the secretary of the VA of our precautionary readiness actions.

Paul's team operated the VHA Emergency Operations Center located on the campus of the Martinsburg, West Virginia, VHA Medical Center. The sprawling Martinsburg campus is a former US Army hospital base covered with parking lots surrounding the main facility and includes multiple free-standing additional buildings. The surface lots behind the hospital is filled with vehicles used in executing emergency response capabilities around the nation. VHA prepositions emergency response materials to include caches of pharmaceutical supplies and response vehicles in various geographically dispersed medical centers under OEM's direction and routinely activates and tests these capabilities. These materials are positioned to reduce the response time to a request from an elected state governor or another federal agency. There are more than 400 wheeled vehicles prepositioned to support the VHA's fourth mission. These vehicles include mobile treatment units, hospital units, command and satellite communication vehicles, mobile generators, tractor trailer units converted into pharmacies, and mobile feeding units operated by the VA Canteen Service.

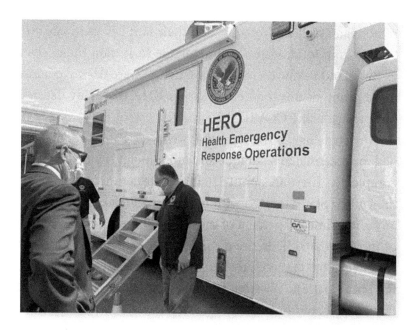

P3: "HERO" command vehicle. Part of the Office of Emergency Management vehicles

Within Dr. Kim's headquarters located in a one-story, no longer operational hospital building on the Martinsburg campus are operations and logistics specialists, planners, engineers, weather forecasters, and FEMA-certified incident management personnel that can be embedded with FEMA anywhere during a disaster to represent VA's interests and offer its capabilities. Each of these specialists is focused on our ability to execute all of VHA's four missions and exercise the agility necessary to support Americas Veterans. In just one of the thousands of examples, after Hurricane Maria struck Puerto Rico in 2017, these emergency management personnel and local VA medical center emergency response personnel hiked on foot for up to a week to reach Veterans who were trapped and ensure all remote and isolated Veterans and their families were safe and had enough food, water, and medicine to sustain themselves as the island roadways and infrastructure were destroyed; one more group of unsung heroes across VHA that truly deserve our praise during COVID-19.

The challenge of the virus that we faced, Paul related to me, had the potential to be unique and monumental in its scope and complexity. There are about 920,000 acute care hospital beds in the United States located within more than 6,000 hospitals. At any given time, 80 percent of those beds, or more than 720,000 of those hospital beds, are occupied with patients. That leaves less than 200,000 acute care beds available for ill patients across the entire nation. We were facing a virus that we believed (at that time) could potentially infect 5 percent of the American population of 332 million. To complete the math, that would indicate that as many as 16.6 million Americans could soon be infected. If 10 percent of those infected needed admission to a hospital, that would require 1.66 million hospital beds. Even if we increased available hospital beds by stopping elective pro-cedures, the likelihood of running out of hospital beds across the entire nation was overwhelmingly likely.

It bears some attention, and I would be remiss to fail to point out that creating operational hospital beds that are staffed with competent personnel and integrated into logistics supply systems is very difficult, even on a routine day unchallenged by a rapidly evolving pandemic. Generally speaking, when a staff member calls out of work, or a key supply or piece of equip-ment is unavailable, another person is called in, or the patient's procedure is shifted to another day. In an emergency, a patient can be transported to another facility, or a less urgent patient can be delayed until supplies and personnel are available. Most hospitals do not have a substantial amount of "surge" capacity, as it is extremely expensive to keep physicians and nurses just "sitting around" or beds that cost tens of thousands of dollars to build and equip empty. There are likely hospitals in your community right now that are operating at more than 90 percent capacity because that is how they keep their doors open and maintain financial viability. The prospect of treating millions of people becoming sick at the same time is quite simply impossible in our existing health care model (and that's just beds and personnel, not yet addressing our "just-in-time" supply chain. More on that topic later.) We were facing a possible scenario where sick Americans would just not have care available.

Success, even in our VHA response, would depend on mitigation of the rate or rapidity of spread of the infection. If we did not slow the spread of the virus, the nation would run out of hospital beds, have nowhere to refer people, and face the potential of massive deaths of patients unable to access care. Even if we planned and executed perfectly, we were still going to have problems with the number and distribution of available beds across the nation for reasons that will become obvious.

As an added complication, not all hospital beds are created equal. The next level of planning was breaking out the types of hospital beds available, and we learned that of those 920,000 acute care beds, there were less than 100,000 intensive care unit (ICU) beds in the US and at any given time, only about 10 percent of those are empty and available.[11] If 10 percent of those anticipated COVID-19 patients were to be admitted to the hospital (1.6 million) and need ICU care, the resultant need could exceed 160,000 admissions for those 10,000 available beds. These numbers were developing and being refined continuously based upon what we knew of the infectiousness and severity of the virus on the populations in other countries. We also began tracking the average number of days a COVID-19-infected ICU patient would need to remain in an ICU in order to predict the impending shortfall of these type of beds. Our Office of Emergency Management and public health teams at the VHA began daily predictions of the potential locations and severity of impending US hospital bed shortages. We further attempted to predict material and personnel shortages in the civilian healthcare sector. Unfortunately, we soon discovered that many of those available (unoccupied) civilian hospital beds were not actually staffed by personnel in the civilian sector. VA as the "backstop" for the nation's health care system was about to be tested.

Within VA, we were facing the following realities:

- VHA operates 8000 acute care medical beds in 175 locations. At any given time, about 85 percent of those beds are filled with patients.

- That left about 1200 empty beds available to dedicate for the COVID-19 response across the nation.

- VHA also operates 8000 long-term (skilled nursing home) care beds and 8000 domiciliary beds for homeless and substance abuse patients.

- In total, we had 24,000 beds, but most were not available. The challenge was to figure out how a system the size of VHA could become an effective backstop for the entire American health care system **when our acute care entire capacity did not meet even 1 percent of the**

anticipated potential need of the American people during the pandemic.

The potential task and possible demand for care appeared to be overwhelming.

I have always operated under a very simple principle: *God gives me the stability of today to prepare for the chaos of tomorrow.* Whatever window I was given, I had to use every possible second that we had to prepare VHA for whatever the American people might need and to fulfill as much of the emerging need as possible.

Sleep became an extraordinarily rare commodity for the VHA leadership team at all levels as the challenge seemed to grow each day. We entered a period during January and February 2020 focused on the observation of the behavior of the virus in other countries, and we utilized that data to attempt to predict the potential size of our own response. We aligned those estimates to the number of patients beginning to emerge across individual states. We found that we had to break each state down to their individual counties and then map the closest VHA hospital facility against the potential need. As we did this, it became very clear that we had to create more acute care beds as quickly as possible but also needed to focus our response on a subset of the potentially very critically ill patients. All this had to occur while ensuring that no Veteran would be denied care while we supported potential civilian non-Veteran patients.

(Author's note: Veteran healthcare is built on a byzantine set of laws and regulations determining who among Veterans and their family members are actually eligible for certain types of VHA provided or paid for health care. Most Veterans have retired or left the uniformed military. But, as noted previously, only about half of America's Veterans were enrolled in VHA healthcare during this time. The other half of Veterans primarily use employer-provided health care insurance and receive care in commercial hospitals. It is important to understand that an unenrolled Veteran can't just "show up" at a VA hospital and receive care under routine, non-emergency circumstances. To avoid confusion in the following pages, I use the term civilian simply to mean anyone not eligible for VA healthcare under routine circumstances, and the term Veteran generally means anyone who is eligible and enrolled for VHA care. The COVID-19 pandemic blurred these lines considerably, as I will discuss in great length. All of that to say, I am not an attorney, nor am I an expert on VA healthcare eligibility except as it impacted my ability to provide care to those in need. One of our concerns was that unenrolled Veterans, when faced with overwhelmed civilian hospitals, would seek care in the VHA. The potential for being overwhelmed within the VHA increased exponentially as we attempted to plan for these contingencies.)

The VHA health care delivery system is divided into eighteen geographic regions known as Veteran Integrated Service Networks (VISNs). Each is led by a VISN Senior Executive Service (SES) director. These directors are highly experienced and universally understand their mission well. They also are highly competitive with each other, and this drives system performance toward improvement to whatever metric we may choose to highlight. I was blessed during this time with an extraordinarily talented operations leader in Renee Oshinski, who served as the assistant under secretary for operations. This position is the senior operations officer of the VHA. Renee had come from the Chicago area VISN 12 leadership position to assume the position of deputy chief of operations from January

2019 to March 2020 and, fortunately for all of us, began her role as the chief operations officer (COO) in March 2020 just as the pandemic accelerated.

Renee was an experienced, thoughtful, and very direct speaking leader with excellent financial and operational performance skills and was well respected by the eighteen regional VISN leaders. Her most significant skill, however, was a willingness to speak truth to power, which would become immensely valuable as we moved the organization forward through the next two years. She was hardened and tested by the shared leadership experience of the 2014 access to care crisis in the Phoenix, Arizona medical center when VHA was accused of allowing Veterans to die on wait lists for care and then covering up the existence of those wait lists. The emotional scars of those events had affected every operational leader across the VHA, no matter where they served. From December 2016 to January 2019, Renee also successfully led the VISN 12 regional system through a crisis in Tomah, Wisconsin, where a single provider inappropriately prescribed large amounts of narcotics to Veterans. This resulted in a series of media articles nicknaming the Tomah facility "Candy Land." (While not germane to the rest of this story, these crises shaped VHA into what it had become when the pandemic started, often resulting in dramatically reduced trust among both Veterans and our congressional oversight partners. The aftereffects of these incidents were what I thought my primary focus would be upon being selected for this job.

Renee had endured an era of senior VHA leaders above her who spread blame to their subordinates and accepted little responsibility themselves. The result was a group of field operational leaders in the medical centers and VISNs less willing to take risk because failure was not tolerated and dealt with operational problems in a very public and punitive manner. This is one of the most important messages of this book: **Crises that challenge a large organization require risk-taking on the part of leaders.** By definition, a crisis is not an everyday challenge. A leader will not be able to predict every outcome of a problem or the success of a proposed solution. Nor will that leader have every bit of information they need before being required to make a decision. Therefore, in order to be successful, leaders must make decisions that have inherent risk. We were not going to know everything about how the virus was going to affect the American population, our Veteran patients, or our facilities and our staff before we needed to act. Waiting for the perfect and fully vetted solution to present itself was not an option. Making decisions, recognizing mistakes, and adapting was, but that requires a level of intestinal fortitude uncommon in government bureaucracy in my experience.

The punitive management culture from which the VHA was emerging reduced the willingness of leaders to take the necessary risk required. Punitive leaders at senior levels stall their organizations while reducing their subordinates' ability to innovate and provide agile solutions to unique challenges. Punitive leaders also deny themselves the intellectual talent and input of their subordinates. Individuals will just not speak truth to power if they are met with demeaning and punitive responses. They will also hide bad news in order to protect their positions in the face of punitive leaders.

Since I had arrived at VHA in July 2018, one of my primary leadership goals was to create followership in my senior leaders and demonstrate that a new culture had arrived. Employees will follow leaders who are reliable and predictable in their responses to problems. By this, I mean that my responses to difficult issues should be predictable, calm, and stable. Each of us will trust those leaders who possess the qualities of predictable responses, honesty, understanding, and recognition. I firmly believe that almost all employees arrive at their work each day wanting to do the right thing. Outcomes sometimes are not what we would like, but those above us on the organizational hierarchy must acknowledge in a positive manner honest and diligent effort. My colleague and longtime friend Rosemary Williams would say that "honest mistakes are always forgiven."

There is a concept called "High Reliability" in organizational performance that is central to developing this cultural transformation. High reliability or zero-defect culture arose in the nuclear power generation industry after the Three Mile Island nuclear accident in March 1979. It also is part of Naval nuclear propulsion, aircraft cockpit operations, and aircraft design. This culture allows the United States Navy to safely operate about 160 nuclear propulsion reactors and without serious accident for decades.

I would ask the reader to think about the organizations that you interact with on a regular or even intermittent basis. There are those who just stand out as organizations that are easy to deal with and "reliable." For me, the United States Army was an organization that asked a lot from me and my family but always was there to support me or my family when I needed help.

As another, USAA insurance focuses its products on uniformed military, Veterans, and families of those who have served. This company handles all of my family's insurance needs. I have personally met a USAA employee only once in almost thirty years of dealing with this company. All my interactions with them are by telephone or more commonly on the internet. Without fail, they have resolved my problem and have reduced what could be very stressful life events. Those events included when my then sixteen-year-old son collided with a Porsche on the day he received his driver's license. Our jeep was fine, my son and the other driver were fine, but the Porsche? Not so much. USAA took this "crisis" and made it manageable, reducing stress, and allowing us to focus on our family instead of their processes or bureaucracy. They have demonstrated consistent reliability.

Reliability engenders trust because process outcomes are predictable. I ask that you consider two pilots arriving for a commercial flight. They may have never met or worked together previously, but aircraft flight operations have become so standardized that they can work through their lack of personal familiarity because their processes and responses to routine and even emergency situations are absolutely routinized. Moving to predictable and routine responses engenders trust in all of us. Only through reliable outcomes of processes will Veterans trust the VHA or any other healthcare provider due to the highly personalized and intimate nature of the work we as medical care providers are called upon to provide.

Moving an organization away from punitive leadership and engendering trust are the foundation of innovation, agility, and the encouragement of leaders to take risks. Renee Oshinski was essential in understanding the emotional investment of our field leaders, and she was brutally honest when I pushed them beyond their comfort zone to prepare the organization for what was about to overwhelm us. Never did she disagree with the direction we were taking, but the ability to reach that goal was substantially enabled by the trusted and honest operational leader that she embodied. Leaders: I cannot overstate Renee's impact on our ability to save lives. If you don't have someone in that "COO" role who sounds like her, I implore you to consider your ability to truly reach your organization's goals and be successful.

In no way could the VHA have responded with the agility the agency demonstrated without the progress we had made in high reliability cultural transformation during the eighteen months I led the VHA prior to the pandemic. That reliability reduces errors, reduces patient harm events, and most importantly, encourages active participation from all leaders and individual team members in problem-solving. These skills would become essential to our response to the complex challenges we were about to face.

CHAPTER FOUR

And So It Begins

THE FIRST CASE OF COVID-19 in the United States was diagnosed on the 20th of January 2020 in a patient admitted to a hospital in the state of Washington. That patient had traveled to Wuhan, China, and returned on the 15th of January. The World Health Organization (WHO) had announced a unique new pneumonia in China on the 9th of January. This announcement occurred twenty-eight days following the December 12th document released from the Wuhan Health minister previously referenced. [12]

Planning at VHA was already underway based on Paul Kim's communication with me over the December holidays. We had begun by assuring the readiness of our equipment and reviewing and validating our stockpiles of medications and materials in order to prepare for any possible future challenge. This required a robust and effective method of being able to "see" available and unoccupied hospital beds to include medical and surgical beds (aka "med surg" beds) and ICU beds. The ability to see available beds had to extend across all levels of the medical centers, the regional VISN networks, and provide national leadership a common and transparent management platform from which to plan future care delivery. One of Renee's primary missions when she served as the deputy chief of operations had been to improve the VHA's bed management system. She delivered an information system in March 2020 as she assumed the role of COO that was profoundly improved from what she had inherited. This system would continue to both improve and be essential throughout our pandemic response.

We had, within the leadership team, established an aspirational goal of creating 4,000 new acute care beds within existing VHA hospitals as quickly as we could, should the spread to the United States not be contained, with an aspirational goal of 50 percent expansion from our pre-pandemic acute care bed capacity to be accomplished over a period of weeks. These beds would need to be equipped and staffed before bringing them online for use. We activated our fourth mission emergency response teams across the nation, and the Martinsburg OEM team established their emergency operations staffing plan. This was also a trigger for each hospital in an at-risk catchment area to activate their own in-house emergency operations centers. In all previous activations, we brought the national emergency response personnel to Washington, DC, from Martinsburg, West Virginia. In this case, we made the decision to leave the emergency response personnel in Martinsburg to reduce the congregation of leadership personnel in a single site and reduce the risk to ongoing emergency operations should COVID-19 infect the team. This would create a leadership redundancy that would protect continuing operations should the leadership team in DC or Martinsburg need to be quarantined.

Coincident to this, we began examining on a daily basis the worldwide chronology of events, including Chinese government responses and the effect of the virus on the Wuhan health care system. We found the Chinese data increasingly difficult to interpret and quickly questioned the accuracy of the data being released. In response, we engaged McKinsey and Company, a global health care consulting firm, in an effort to provide reliable daily data on what was happening in countries around the world with this disease. McKinsey not only had offices around the world. Many of these offices were staffed with international health care teams. McKinsey had begun producing daily publicly available updates on disease progression and health system responses. Johns Hopkins University had also begun producing data on the worldwide and US pandemic spread. We wanted to ensure we had actual human intelligence gatherers on the ground in various countries, and, therefore, we engaged this team of experts to support our internal US-based team.

VHA has robust data analytic capability, and our inhouse team was initially promoting the use of COVID-19-caused patient deaths as an indicator of future work volume. I rejected this proposal as I believed the death rate was a lagging indicator of future severe disease propagation and would not allow us to quickly assess and develop response plans to what might happen in the weeks ahead. We desperately needed to literally see the future. The McKinsey team was led by Scott Blackburn, a former VA deputy secretary and Veteran who I had worked with under the Obama administration. Scott understood the VHA and sheer size of its operating systems. Scott and his team were invaluable in providing timely data on the challenges that would face us. McKinsey also provided Gretchen Berlin, a senior partner and highly experienced leader, in system transformation. These two leaders accepted every challenge and provided robust counsel to the VHA leadership team as we developed our response plan.

My instructions to Gretchen, Scott, and their team was that we needed to see the future. I wanted to see demand for COVID-19-related care two weeks into the future. I wanted to know what might happen to the nation and at VHA in order to give us time to move the organization to where our hospitalization capacity needed to be. I wanted to understand what the prevalence of the disease would be, meaning what percent of the population would become infected at the county level. Of those infected, what percent of those would need hospitalization, what percent of those hospitalized would need ICU services, and finally, what percent would die? These were unreasonable questions in the initial phases of the pandemic, but we were seeing elected state and local officials asking for support based on possible worst-case scenarios that would be impossible to sustain across the entirety of the nation. In addition, we needed to understand what the effect of the virus was on health care workers. Could we sustain the VHA workforce? How much did we need to grow the workforce to sustain the current VHA delivery system plus an additional 4000 acute care beds? Would we lose 10 percent of our workforce to quarantine, infection, and hospitalization like some nations had?[13] These questions must be answered. And they needed to be answered as quickly as possible.

This VHA workforce was going into battle to support the victims of this new and mostly unknown disease. We needed to understand how to sustain the mission. Until we understood potential losses of available personnel, we were blind as to how to staff the system.

Our active engagement in fourth mission emergency management activities began as cruise ship passengers were brought to US military bases in order to quarantine on the 9th of March

2020. Four military bases were used to quarantine passengers, and VHA deployed personnel to support any enrolled or unenrolled Veterans among the group of passengers sequestered during a CDC-proposed fourteen-day quarantine. As a planning consideration, we determined that there were 314 passenger-occupied cruise ships afloat and in use in the world with a capacity of just under 600,000 passengers and staff. Not all of them would come to the United States, but we were concerned that if this model was followed, more than 200,000 Americans might need to be housed for quarantine on military bases. The idea of housing all those who were even scheduled to dock at US ports in the next month consumed the Department of Defense's initial response planning. We began to be concerned that the DOD would have little capacity left to give when the pandemic really began to spread across the rest of the nation's population, and we moved from quarantine of those exposed to actual COVID-19 patient care. (Cruise ships, their capacity, and how to evacuate and quarantine their passengers were certainly not something I thought I would ever have to know about when I started this job.)

VHA's mission in support of DOD was to support those Veterans exiting the cruise ships and sustain their medications and care while quarantined, thus unloading at least those Veteran patients from DOD medical care responsibility. This is a routine mission for the VHA and is similar to our pre- and post-hurricane support when many Veterans are separated from their medications and need support for ongoing health challenges, such as diabetes, hypertension, long-term oxygen use, or even end-stage renal disease, including the need for dialysis. Volunteer personnel from across the nation were adequate for this initial mission and deployed as part of our standard emergency operations to involved military bases. By the very nature of this mission, these personnel were sent to coastal communities and followed our "traditional" model of sending people from unaffected areas to those areas impacted. This mission dominated the news for weeks, and for many national leaders, it became a "shiny object" on which to focus, often ignoring the rapidly emerging problem of protecting the rest of the nation.

Already, by the 1st of March, while we were preparing to execute the quarantine mission on military bases, the disease had, however, already spread across the country to New York City. The virus had grown exponentially, and by March 11, just two days after starting the DOD quarantine mission, COVID-19-infected patients in New York were five times greater than the entire remainder of the United States. In fact, one-third of US cases were in New York.[14] New York government leaders, from the governor to the New York City health commissioner, were asking the same questions we had been asking since January. How many cases would there be? What percent of those would be sick enough to need hospitalization? How many would need ICUs, and how many would die? Could the health care workforce be protected, and would that workforce continue to come to work if the city around them and their own families were overcome with disease?

I believe some of the key errors in the US national response were made during this period by politicians ignoring the public health community, failing to directly engage with health care delivery systems, or responding to fearmongering perpetuated by political leaders and the media.

In combat, we actually have a term for this period. It is referred to as "the fog of war." It was exactly the reason we had asked the McKinsey team to "see" the future. We had been working in VHA for weeks to narrow this "fog" as much as possible. Almost all the volume predictions of possible future care that would be required was based on disease prevalence predictions (how much of the American population would become infected). Subtle changes from 5 percent to 6 percent in the number of infected individuals in a community would dramatically change the amount of care that would possibly be needed. In addition, the rapidity of spread, what we called the R0, (pronounced "R naught") reflects how contagious an infectious agent is. A number greater than one indicates that for every infected person, they will infect more than one person around them. We have recently seen R0 over 7 for the omicron variant, thus the incredible spread across the population with each infected person infecting seven others.[15] All this was unknown early in the pandemic, and my impression was that the New York state government leadership had chosen to promote a worst-case scenario that was not sustainable across the American health care system's response. They didn't know what would happen, so they just asked for everything with minimal context or proper public health planning.

This was a once-in-a-hundred-year event. For those in positions of leadership untrained in military or crisis response, there was significant anxiety, and there was fear. Few had the counsel of a Paul Kim, Renee Oshinski, or the McKinsey team to rely on. Few health or political leaders in city or state government were trained for a crisis that would cost more than a million lives. Their response was simply, "Give us everything" for a worst-case scenario. For generations, all responses in military planning for war requires balance and preservation of assets for future yet unknown contingencies. There is a profound difference between this type of wartime contingency planning and the political responses that ultimately focus on risk avoidance by leaders ill-prepared for a rapidly evolving crisis. In addition, this emerging catastrophe was entirely different from a post-event (for example, hurricane) response, as the challenges were unfolding with each passing hour and day. The nation was in the middle of a fight not seen for one hundred years.

These worst-case planning factors pushed those state level leaders in positions of power to call on their governors and ask for a massive influx of ventilators, nurses, and hospital beds. Hospitals in NYC and portions of New Jersey were overwhelmed, but the response that followed created a nationwide model of flooding massive assets into a community that nearly every governor and mayor eventually wanted to be repeated across the country. This early model of deployment wasted valuable assets by placing them where they were not going to be needed or brought more assets to the community than could possibly be employed in direct patient care. The decision to engage in conversion of conference centers or exposition halls into massive hospital bed facilities was an example of this. My impression is that those sites were able to care only for very low acuity level patients, basically, patients who were not very ill. Their ability to care for, sustain, and then provide continuity of care for the sickest patient in this type of pandemic response was just not possible.

Just consider the difficulty in recording and memorializing care delivered for very sick patients who are going to need long-term support. For most of these converted centers, there was no electronic medical record system. There was no system to move laboratory results to the bedside; it was all performed by hand. The ability to logistically resupply such a facility once the initial push pack of consumable materials was expended was going to be very difficult to execute and sustain. Those politicians that decided to establish these pop-up hospitals failed to recognize the sheer complexity of today's hospital operations and the complexity of care required for patients with severe COVID-19. There seemed to be an impression that all COVID-19 patients would be the same and, therefore, they just needed more space and more beds. Without proper triage, these facilities were not only potentially ineffective but could have been dangerous.

In response to requests from the state and local governments, NYC was flooded with federal government assets to include the Navy hospital ship, the USS Comfort, with more than 1200 hospital personnel that arrived on March 30. In addition, 1000 federal medical workers were deployed by early April. Most of these were US Public Health Service (USPHS) uniformed health workers. The USPHS only has about six thousand health workers nationwide, and more than 15 percent of them were in New York. In addition, 2,700 New York National Guard soldiers were activated by the New York governor. In addition, field hospitals were established in high-risk areas, including parks.[16]

When the USS Comfort arrived, there were 36,200 cases of COVID-19 in NYC. The governor and mayor of NYC announced, "The worst is yet to come." Over the next few weeks, the Comfort would treat only 179 patients, and by the 21st of April, three weeks after arrival, the governor announced the ship was no longer needed. It left NYC on the 30th of April.[17] The remaining patients on the USS Comfort were moved to VA hospitals in Manhattan and the Bronx. [18]

This massive mobilization and deployment drained available personnel from other future responses. My view of these events was that the president, in good faith, responded to the loudest voice, which was the then governor of New York. Temporary hospitals, however, are very difficult to sustain except for treatment of the least ill patient who, by definition, consumes low levels of resources. Highly trained and competent health-related personnel are difficult to sustain for prolonged periods of time in these facilities, and logistics resupply are effective only with the support of trained military health logisticians. Future pandemic response should emphasize a model of collocation of these care delivery expansion assets to existing hospital infrastructure to unload all extraneous demands on the highly experienced health delivery personnel within an existing facility and allow those civilian hospitals to focus on the most critically ill patients. The model VHA would follow throughout this time was the expansion and conversion of VA medical centers. This would include conversion of surface and multilevel parking structures on hospital campuses into care delivery locations of various levels of intensity.

The nation's response should have recognized that caring for the minimally or even moderately ill is a dramatically simpler process than pulmonary critical care medicine with all the comorbid complications of a COVID-19 patient. Ideally, hospitals and ICUs should orient to the critically ill and, therefore, most complex demands of ill patients in order to **"Save every life you can."**

I have used the above quotation throughout this manuscript and in the title. As VHA leaders around the country began to realize the enormity of the challenge they faced, we met in a daily system wide operations center meeting. A number of VISN leaders questioned if they could sustain the effort and meet the needs of both Veterans and civilians. My response was based on my clinical and wartime combat service. My direction to all clinicians and leaders was to recognize that being "all in" during combat means we will wisely use every asset and consume as many resources as necessary and available in order to save every life we possibly could. We would leave nothing on the table, no stone unturned. Our skill in critical care and our experience in caring for combat-wounded Veterans prepared us for what was to come.

Austerity in combat-related healthcare is practiced and trained across all branches of the military health care delivery system. While deployed to Afghanistan and during high casualty flow for coalition and American service members, I needed to make tough and gut-wrenching decisions. I was empowered to accept injured Afghan adults and children to our care system during my deployment to Bagram, but there was one caveat: In no circumstance could care for those Afghan patients preclude the availability of care for an American or coalition service member ill or injured in combat operations. There was a daily review of our available beds, blood, and supplies and alignment of those materials to anticipated combat operations and expected casualty flow. Unfortunately, this required that I keep a mental note of which foreign national would be removed from support should an American or coalition service member need help. I prayed that I would never need to make those decisions.

I exercised that mental list only once and will be forever indebted to the collocated Egyptian military hospital and its commander for accepting those patients and ensuring their continued care. I was forced to limit the use of blood products to coalition forces after a particularly horrendous bombing of an Afghan school by the enemy and the coincident spoilage of blood resupply from Europe during transport. The school that was bombed had been named after Afghan President Karzai's father in Kandahar in southern Afghanistan, making it a target for the Taliban. The Taliban warned that the school must be shut down. When it was not, they blew up the school with well over 100 children inside. We accepted twenty-three of the most critically injured children, all victims of the bombing. Even the most hardened of our trauma delivery staff were overwhelmed with grief as they cared for and attempted to save the lives of as many of these innocent children as they could.

As the hours passed, it became more and more clear to me that our blood supply was critically low and would likely run out. Faced with a reality no one would ever choose, I made the toughest decision of my life and ordered that no more transfusions would be given to the children to maintain our supply for potential US casualties. Understandably, this decision was not well received by my hospital personnel.

That night, I decided to walk the halls of the hospital about 3 am. As I rounded a corner of a connecting hallway, I encountered a line of US medical soldiers waiting to donate blood. They all looked at me, and I said nothing. Nothing needed to be said, but I was forever grateful that children's lives were saved by the selfless acts of those medical soldiers who donated their own blood to save every life they could. Heroism is often very quiet.

I experienced this same quiet heroism and resolute commitment to mission over and over from virtually every VHA employee throughout the pandemic. They did not falter, even when exhausted or when one of their fellow care givers was lost to this wretched virus.

The ability to sustain hope is essential in all human challenges, but it is most important to those receiving health care. Think of those around you battling life-threatening illness or

injury and the obvious need for hope of recovery in order to bol-
ster their willingness to continue the exhausting fight. The presence of hope is also essential to all of those actually delivering
health care. Even in end-of-life or hospice care, the presence of
hope is centered on delivering reduced pain and the respectful
care support that all of us hope to receive even when the outcome is apparent, unavoidable, and imminent. This is also the
basis of health care delivery in combat and a model for what I
hoped to achieve in leading VHA during the COVID-19 fight.

Managing austere medical assets (both material and personnel) through the early stages of the pandemic needed the
expertise of competent and experienced operational health
leaders who understood how complex and dangerous this
evolving pandemic could possibly become.

CHAPTER FIVE

Ensuring Care Is Available

OUR NATION'S SOLDIERS, SAILORS, airmen, and Marines will sacrifice and perform heroic acts of bravery if they believe their sacrifice is respected by their leaders and their fellow citizens. These acts will occur only if they are convinced their sacrifice is both needed and, in some way, recognized. Part of that recognition and a demonstration of the value of their service is the provision of collocated and readily available health care to provide support for warriors if they are injured or become ill during their mission activities. In World War One, if a service member was combat-wounded, over 26 percent died of their wounds. (204,000 wounded, 53,402 died of their wounds). There were an additional 63,114 non-combat deaths due to disease in the American Army during this time to include thirty thousand killed by the influenza pandemic. [19] During WWII, the survival rate of the wounded had changed little from previous wars. Dramatic improvement in wounded survival in more recent conflicts reflects significant advances in trauma and resuscitation care by military health professionals. This improvement was primarily because of advances in combat-related health care delivery and emerging germ theory (tools to fight infection). This eventually resulted in the need for complex rehabilitation services for service members surviving their wounds, which has only grown as our field-delivered combat medicine has improved during war.

The work of General Omar Bradley, when assigned at the end of WWII as the leader of the VA, was based upon bringing America's most advanced healthcare and rehabilitation specialists to the care of the recovering wounded. He believed that excellence in rehabilitative care could only be accomplished by collocating VA hospitals with the major academic medical centers around the United States. The resultant delivery system seventy-five years later is foundationally based upon 1,700 academic affiliations between VHA hospitals and nearly every academic medical center in the nation. In many cities, VA medical centers are literally connected by bridges and walkways to many premier medical centers and medical schools. The medical staff of these medical centers boasts the combined credentialling of VHA providers in both systems. This creates the availability of America's most advanced care providers for the benefit of this countries Veterans.[20]

I found myself in the spring of 2020 in the same position I experienced in Afghanistan in dealing with the need for austerity throughout the pandemic. Unlike in combat where the ethics and norms of warfare provided guidelines for my decisions, during the pandemic, the political overlay of available capabilities and assets being moved by nonoperational (elected or appointed political) "experts" complicated the response. It reminded me of stories of President Lyndon Johnson standing over a map of Vietnam in the White House, deciding where troops would deploy. There must always be deference by political leaders to subject matter operational expertise in decisions on health asset utilization during this type of national crisis response. Although I am respectful of the role of elected leaders in fulfilling the wishes of the American people, complex care delivery operational decisions during a crisis should respect the role of those with true crisis management and medical response expertise. In situations like this, I have found I have increasingly little tolerance for politically-motivated decisions and the interference of those with political or salacious agendas, such as the media. I continue to respect and appreciate the oversight as provided by congressional oversight committees in judging how well we performed, but effective execution of immediate crisis decisions should be left with the operational SMEs with health care delivery expertise. (I ask the reader to refer back to my experience during my first night in Afghanistan, related earlier.)

We found ourselves with much of the nation's federal response, both uniformed and civilian, deployed too early in the pandemic response to areas challenged but not completely overwhelmed. This occurred before we actually knew the location and severity of the enemy we faced. The Department of Defense was the primary recipient of executing these requests, but in order to meet these deployments in support of state requests, the DOD medical care delivery system was forced to reduce routine care to service members and their families, and in order to meet their health care needs, it had to increase the purchase of care in communities already overloaded by COVID-19 escalating demand. These decisions reduced needed uniformed medical personnel in DOD-staffed facilities. This also left DOD personnel assigned to pop-up facilities in communities with few patients, thus wasting critical, highly competent expertise in the response.

This was not just a profound waste of resources; it also left VHA in an even more vulnerable position as DOD assets and USPHS assets were committed and expended. As we grew the available VHA hospital beds across the nation during the period of January to March 2020, we recognized that there was significant risk to ensuring the continued access to care for our enrolled Veterans. We also recognized that many of the unenrolled Veterans across the United States would choose VA should access to care in the civilian sector or at DOD become compromised and unavailable. We all agreed that we could not place Veterans at risk while exercising any possible fourth mission. It also became apparent that we would be able to successfully reach our available bed growth from a pre-pandemic level of 8,000 to as many as 12,000 acute care beds. This 50-percent inpatient bed capacity growth had been left entirely up to our medical center and VISN directors, and while we centrally tracked and supported progress, we deferred the distribution of beds to the operations experts who understood the availability of personnel and supplies at each facility.

Staffing these new beds would come from two areas, the first being newly hired government personnel. We pledged to remove many of the barriers to hiring employees into a VHA job. Prior to the pandemic, the average VHA professional nurse hire would take at least 120 days. We vowed to cut that time to three days. Only through rapid hiring could we compete with commercial health systems for available talent. This was accomplished with the extraordinary support of VA and VHA human resources assets as well as the federal government Office of Personnel Management (OPM), who designed a fundamentally new model for federal hiring that allowed us to compete effectively for healthcare talent across multiple markets. I cannot overemphasize the role of VHA Workforce Management led by Jessica Bonjorni and her team and their relationships with the federal government HR experts at OPM, who made the impossible possible at this critical time. These were consummate professionals who transformed government hiring in a few weeks. We also were able to financially incentivize our workforce to stay with us and volunteer for fourth mission deployments through bonuses and other awards, bearing in mind the need to prevent depletion of the workforce within any at-risk geographic areas.

The concept of "supported" and "supporting" VISNs developed as we contemplated massive personnel moves across the nation. The operational concept was that an individual region that was hard hit by COVID-19 patients was *supported* by another VISN or region that was not as challenged. This operating concept is organic to the military and referred to as operational and strategic reserves whose power can be moved as necessary to influence the outcome of an engagement.

The second method to enhance available personnel would come from shifting ambulatory care staffing as COVID-19 cases began to elevate in a region. We found that ambulatory care delivered face to face with patients in these areas of COVID-19 escalation fell off dramatically as patients feared exposure to the COVID-19 virus. We, therefore, found that we could reduce our ambulatory care staffing and repurposed and retrained thousands of ambulatory care nurses in order to support our critical care inpatient nursing teams. On any given day, VHA performs about two hundred thousand ambulatory visits utilizing a workforce that is purely dedicated to the ambulatory care mission.[21] Unlike most other health care systems, VHA employs a large number of ambulatory care professional nurses in support of that operation.

VISN 12 in the upper Midwest designed an eighteen-hour training program to enhance the critical care skills of an ambulatory care nurse in order to support an ICU care delivery team as we repurposed those ambulatory care nurses to inpatient work. Every VISN created a similar model to enhance critical care depth. We recognized that this training did not develop a fully-qualified critical care nurse, but it did allow a critical care nurse to arrive at work knowing that they were not alone. This was also occurring as family visitations to hospitals were suspended. The care of patients without their family's presence at the bedside created a huge emotional burden for even experienced critical care personnel. Creating the availability of a hand to hold as life slipped away from a critically ill patient was as important as any complex care we delivered. We could not expect the critical care team to sustain itself through this protracted and intense response without support, and I am proud we were able to innovate quickly to provide it. I am also incredibly proud of the thousands of nurses who took on this difficult role.

This was no different than my experience many years before with trauma teams faced with massive potential pediatric deaths. The presence of additional personnel to provide care would sustain the workforce through some horrific challenges and lonely shifts of care. Care was also complicated during this challenge by our VHA no-visitor policy, which, although well-intentioned to protect patients, personnel, and visitors from virus spread, it actually created additional demands on the workforce to communicate with family, create communication tools for family and patients through electronic devices, and ensure no Veteran was ever alone, even as they passed.

The emotional connection the VHA workforce expresses to Veterans stems from the fact that one-third of VA employees are Veterans themselves. For those who are not, mission commitment arises from the service of their spouses, parents, grandparents, aunts and uncles, brothers and sisters, or their children. That mission commitment connects these extraordinary care providers to their patients in some of the most unique expressions of love and care that I have ever experienced in my over forty years of delivering medical care.

Returning in time to the 31st of January 2020, the first cases of COVID-19 had been diagnosed in Italy. The virus tore through the Italian population, causing the country's leadership to order a nationwide lockdown of its citizens. My future planners and the McKinsey team had become convinced that the Chinese data on COVID-19 had become increasingly (and potentially purposefully) inaccurate or distorted. We had begun looking for other models to see what the American future might look like. We believed that Italy was a transparent society with an independent media. We also believed the Italians possessed a reasonably high-quality health care system. Because of all of this, we believed we could use Italy as a predictive model of what might happen in the United States.

We watched in horror from afar as the Lombardy region of Italy was quickly overwhelmed. Within eight weeks, 16 million Italians were in quarantine; shockingly, a quarter of the sixty million total Italian population. [22] Hospitals were overwhelmed with patients, and health systems began to collapse. We saw reports of ambulance response teams completely sidelined by infection. We also had reports of centralized facility oxygen systems pipes freezing from high oxygen flow, thus collapsing the ability to provide oxygen to critically ill patients. We also had reliable reports of health care workers across the Lombardy region becoming infected and dying at extraordinary rates. As we applied these reports and their data to our future planning, we began to estimate the possibilities for VHA if our workforce became infected at the same rates as the Italian medical workforce. These numbers, when applied to the VHA, predicted a system that was in significant likelihood of failure.

Initial estimates were that as much as 10 percent of our 360,000 employees could be sidelined by COVID-19 in the February and March time frame. We estimated that we would need to hire as many as fifteen thousand employees during each of those two months. As we were watching these international events, there was still almost no data on American health care workers and how they were faring during the initial phases of the pandemic. An exception to this was the Henry Ford Health System in Detroit, which estimated that 10 percent of its workforce had become exposed or infected and was unable to work. This was very similar to Italy. Sustainment of the workforce, therefore, became my number-one priority. In no way could we sustain the newly expanded bed capacity without the expansion of the patient-facing workforce.

We thus recognized that the ability of our system to respond to COVID-19 was completely dependent on a very well-trained, cohesive, and *healthy* nursing workforce. The crisis that appeared to be looming across the world and within the walls of the VHA would only be overcome with professional nurses at the bedside of infected patients delivering what we now realized was very complex care. We needed professional nurses, and we needed them now.

Our employees were seeing the same reports, and fear amongst VHA employees was significant as they recognized that they as frontline workers were at risk, and that risk could extend to their own families. We began to receive reports of employees staying in hotel rooms between shifts to protect their families from possible exposure. We also had multiple reports of families requesting clinical employees change clothes at work or leave their work clothes and shoes outside their homes when they returned from work at the VHA.

The ensuing hiring process brought over eighty-five thousand new employees, many of them professional nurses into the VHA over the next ten months. We met our hiring goals only because OPM and VHA HR were aligned to the crisis that was facing us. We began tracking weekly hiring and discussing challenges openly across the system. Best practices included hiring fairs where offers of employment were made immediately to personnel, and the paperwork would catch up later. If we didn't hire, our sister academic hospital or another community hospital would hire the professional within a day, and we knew it.

I should note that this was a highly controversial effort, as we were waiving or delaying numerous steps in the hiring process that were established over decades of federal hiring, including background checks, fingerprinting, badge issuance, mandatory training, and more. My thoughts at the time were that I would rather have someone on the payroll actively working to deliver care while we got the paperwork caught up than have them go elsewhere. We pledged that if we found any of them unfit to work for us, we would immediately terminate their employment. I still believe that my other alternative was to collapse the system because there was no one to care for the patient. I stand by that decision.

In 2004, John Barry had written a nonfiction book entitled *The Great Influenza: The Story of the Deadliest Plague in History.* [23] This was the story of the 1918 influenza pandemic that had begun in Haskell County, Kansas, and over the next two years, had infected 500 million people worldwide, killing as many as

50 million people around the world. I had read this book when it was published and had kept it in my library because I felt the first seventy-five pages very well summarized the evolution of American medicine into the scientific culture that had evolved since the late 1800s. That pandemic had also brought huge challenges to the health care workforce, and they were starting to sound eerily like what was being reported in places like Italy. During the Great Influenza, there were also significant leadership challenges resulting from political interference in the pandemic response, political interference that was motivated by an effort to maintain the morale of the American people during the early stages of WWI. Part of this involved manipulating the media and influenza infection data that was ultimately hidden from Americans in order to maintain the morale of the public. This significantly underplayed the extent of the 1918 pandemic, obviously with disastrous consequences.

Because of all of the similarities to the COVID-19 pandemic, I asked the entire VHA leadership team, including those in the central office and the VISN leaders in the field, to read or reread this book. Learning from history would hopefully prevent us from repeating the mistakes of the past. The nation would have been well served if more leaders (including political) had read this comprehensive work.

CHAPTER SIX

Negative Pressure Airflow and the Role of the Facility Engineer

FOLLOWING THE NEW YORK governor's model of demanding a massive influx of supplies and personnel based on worst-case planning scenarios, multiple other states followed the same path in requests for support from the federal government. These requests consumed the critical response assets of DOD and USPHS and overwhelmed FEMA, which was handling them. Temporary care centers were erected across the nation with the support of the Army Corps of Engineers. One of the best (worst) examples of this was in Chicago with the conversion of the McCormick Place Convention Center into an alternate care facility with 3,000 beds. The city of Chicago would spend 65 million dollars between March and the end of April on a minimal care hospital that would open and then rapidly close by May, having treated just twenty-nine patients. An additional $15 million was spent on staffing utilizing primarily private medical staffing contractors. There is little information on actual staff assigned to the facility, but one contract reported by the Chicago Sun Times stated that 274 personnel were to be supplied from a firm in Kansas. The hospital opened in mid-April and closed three weeks later (Chicago Sun Times,

Nov 13, 2020).[24] This type of waste was justified by politicians in leadership of the community as, "We acted in an abundance of caution."

Unfortunately, that "abundance of caution" would substantially deprive the medical delivery infrastructure, civilian and federal, from leveraging available assets effectively. The consumption of resources to build, equip, and staff a facility this large is a tremendous demand upon an already stressed system. A supply chain already stressed to meet the demands of a community or region cannot sustain wasted effort such as this. This example is dramatically different than crisis response decision-making that involves risk-taking. The "abundance of caution" model is simply flooding the community with resources with little understanding of the overwhelming secondary effects these (usually political) decisions have on the consumption of scarce resources. These decisions had regional and national implications and reduced the agility of profoundly stressed regional and national supply and personnel health care sustainment systems.

During this time, VHA was in the process of reexamining its infrastructure under the leadership of the VHA senior facility engineer, Ed Litvin. Ed, a graduate of West Virginia University, is a soft-spoken professional who was trained by VHA and has spent his thirty-five-year government career making one of the oldest health care facility infrastructures in the world continue to work. His official title at VHA is Director, Healthcare Environment and Facilities Programs.

Across the nation, the average age of a civilian hospital is reported as about ten and one-half years.[25] At VHA, our hospitals average in excess of fifty-eight years old, with some buildings still in use, reaching more than a hundred years old.[26] The ability to manage advances in data transmission to the patient bedside is a massive challenge for health care providers delivering care in buildings that were constructed decades before computers were even invented. Each year as the president's budget is debated in Congress, the capital investment needs of this aging VHA infrastructure is acknowledged by Congress, but a definitive solution is often blocked by mostly parochial local interests that preserve ancient facilities under the hope that a massive multi-billion dollar building program will replace a hundred-year-old facility. In many of these locations, Veterans have moved away from the community, and the community can no longer justify a facility of the size and capacity that currently exists.

These VHA facilities are often housed on large multiacre federal enclaves similar to a military base; in fact, some are built on shuttered former military enclaves. The original concept one hundred years ago was to provide a quiet place of healing or an asylum-type care delivery model. This resulted in large facilities and massive buildings with their inherent challenges of sustainment. [27]

In response to the challenges of the pandemic, we needed to not only create additional patient care rooms capable of caring for the sickest patients, but we also needed to equip those rooms with what is called "negative pressure" air flow. A negative pressure room ensures that the virus contained in an infected patient's room could not contaminate the rest of the hospital through airborne transmission and would stay in isolated COVID-19-positive areas of the facility. The presence of negative airflow would allow health care operations for routine (uninfected) patients to continue safely even with large numbers of COVID-19 patients. The complexity of the work to ensure negative airflow environments in a facility cannot be overstated. That complexity was complicated by old buildings that Ed's teams across the enterprise of the VHA overcame by creating air outflow often through windows, ceilings, and even newly created fenestrations in exterior walls to ensure environmental safety. Some facilities became a labyrinth of heavy gauge plastic tarps secured across doorways and hallways with industrial fans positioned over openings created in a maze of fenestrations to the outside. As the scientific world debated airborne potential for COVID-19 spread, we made the decision to create as much negative airflow as possible and control the movement of air within as many of our facilities as possible. VHA engineering teams across the country were quickly added to my list of unsung and relatively invisible heroes of this pandemic.

The 8,000 "long-term care" (nursing home) beds that the VHA operates are often physically connected to or within the VHA medical centers' buildings. This colocation allows VHA to staff these facilities with higher levels of professional personnel than virtually any other long-term care provider in the nation. I will discuss the value of this staffing model later, but the collocation, connection, or even the long-term care facility housed within a medical center simplified our ability to control airflow within these facilities, thus allowing control of viral spread. It was becoming increasingly clear at this time that the most vulnerable portion of our Veteran population (and all Americans) were the institutionalized elderly who suffered from multiple debilitating comorbid conditions. The potential death rate from COVID-19 of an elderly Veteran with diabetes, hypertension, and chronic lung disease appeared to be much higher than younger patients without comorbid conditions. For this reason, we approached managing personnel movements from the hospital into and out of the more than 130 VHA extended care living facilities in a purposeful and deliberate manner. In addition, Ed Litvin's engineers approached air movement and the deliberate creation of secure transfer locations for the movement of materials into and out of the long-term care areas of the facility in order to ensure safety of this extremely vulnerable population. As just one example, the ability to deliver a meal to a patient's bedside became a complex and labor-intensive process. The entire process required the engineers and infection control teams to retrain and reconfigure what was, in most cases, congregate meal service in a restaurant-type dining room into bedside individual trays of food delivered to every patient who were then fed alone in their rooms. This change required the ability to deliver over twenty-four thousand individual meals every day to separate rooms. (Pre-pandemic, meal tray delivery was to 130 common congregate dining rooms.)

This separation or, more appropriately, isolation of elderly and infirm patients had huge second and third-order effects on patients' functional capacity. We recognized that patients with cognitive decline were stabilized by visits and conversations with their family and friends. They were also stabilized by the dynamics of the community of patients that they interacted with and dined with each day. As Veterans were isolated in order to reduce the spread of the virus, we began to see substantial decline in cognitive functioning across this patient population. Families observed this also in the reduced verbal ability of their Veteran in-video calls conducted with their family members from our facilities, a devastating blow to an already isolated and challenged population, many of whom were WWII, Korean War, and Vietnam War-era Veterans.

The VHA geriatric and mental health teams worked diligently to create an environment of enhanced human-to-human interaction. Although valiant and persistent in their efforts, I became convinced that all humans (at all ages) need personal face-to-face contact and robust personal interactions. As I watch a generation of Americans spending multiple hours each day in interaction with friends on electronic media utilizing handheld devices, I have become more convinced than ever that interaction in the actual physical presence of others is irreplaceable in the short- and long-term maintenance of cognitive and healthy emotional function.

It should be noted that each VHA medical center has their own on-site engineering department. These engineers also support the long-term care facilities and ambulatory facilities within a regional medical center's catchment area. Ed's team was learning and innovating across the 175 hospitals and more than 130 long-term care facilities to expand negative air flow rooms and corridors as quickly as possible. We rapidly began to recognize in response to this work that isolating the virus was very difficult in any facility. We also realized that employee movement in and out of COVID-19-positive areas created significant risk that needed to be mitigated by the engineers but also by substantial retraining of our entire labor force. Infectious disease prevention retraining became essential, not just for bedside medical personnel but also for maintenance personnel, food service workers, and facility cleaners. This resulted in the need to double the personnel performing any function. Returning to the earlier example of the food tray delivery process, a food service delivery person could only move from the kitchen to the exchange point of COVID-19-negative to positive portions of the hospital. At this point, a second food service employee would need to receive the tray and deliver it to a patient. Every process that delivered value to the COVID-19-positive regions of the facility required this type of duplication, an amazingly difficult toll to sustain.

As an additional complicating factor, VHA is blessed with more than sixty thousand unpaid volunteers, many of them aging Veterans who connect to the Veteran community through volunteering within the medical centers and care delivery system. These volunteers give hundreds of thousands of hours each year to provide a myriad of tasks, including wayfinding in our hospitals and support information desks across virtually every area of the facility. As we closed the facilities to outside visitation, the actual need for these volunteers dissipated overnight. Virtually, the entire volunteer labor force was sidelined as we considered the risk of infection to this volunteer population too great to allow their work to be repurposed for other more direct patient care needs. It was a terribly difficult decision that I recognized had a large impact on some of our most dedicated and friendly supporters. I know bringing them back will mean the world to our facilities and the Veterans they serve.

Coincident to these debates, we needed to create a screening process at the entrances of our buildings in order to ensure those with illness did not unintentionally carry the virus through the hallways and contaminate non COVID-19 areas. We also needed to ensure those possibly infected patients seeking access to care were routed to those areas of the facility most able to safely care for them while reducing staff risk. Those with symptoms were routed through tents and temporary buildings that we erected outside our emergency rooms. Because patients may not realize they were ill, we placed trained screeners at our entrances that questioned and took temperatures in an effort to protect the vulnerable within the medical centers. This became very high-risk work, and many of those who voluntarily took on this work became infected with the virus. Remarkably, virtually all of these "screeners" who had been infected voluntarily returned upon recovery to resume the same work.

In one poignant example, during my medical center travels, I encountered a dentist whose practice had been suspended during the pandemic and had volunteered to work at a medical center front entrance as a screener. He had been infected, recovered, and returned to his temporary job with the confidence that he had acquired natural immunity. The debate over the adequacy of post-infection acquired natural immunity remains one of the profound shortcomings of the work the research community has completed on this virus and its effect on humans. Accurate information on the difference between infection-acquired and vaccine-acquired immunity is confusing to even the infectious disease and public health community. As the nation examines the response to this virus, there is little doubt that understanding the levels of antibodies necessary to protect an individual from infection would have significantly simplified our response and viral prevention processes. Regardless, I was proud of that dentist who took on some of the most dangerous and tiring work in his facility to help keep Veterans and his fellow employees safe, another unsung hero on my list.

CHAPTER SEVEN

When the Impact of a Decision Doesn't Align

As NYC WAS EXPERIENCING rapid increases in the number of active COVID-19 cases reported across the city, we soon recognized the danger of infection in densely inhabited communities. In these areas, the population lived in apartment-style buildings and, in addition, those residing in small multigenerational homes that forced individuals to live in close physical proximity had significant infection risk. The VISN 2 Network Director Joan McInerney, MD, led the NY and New Jersey VHA integrated delivery system. Joan quickly recognized the impending fourth mission the state of New York and NYC would request. As she and I discussed our options to ensure continuing care to ill Veterans while expanding the ability of the VHA system to accept non-Veteran patients, we examined our ability to reduce COVID-19 spread in our VHA buildings as the number of infected patients grew each day. It seemed reasonable as these events emerged that we would congregate our COVID-19 patients from across that hard-hit region at our Manhattan VA Medical Center. This would allow us to maintain COVID-19 negative facilities in other areas and thus protect patients and staff. The Manhattan VA medical center is blessed with very significant critical care talent and was performing highly complex medical interventions in partnership with their academic partners at New York University, Mt Sinai, NY Medical College, SUNY Health Science Center, and others. Joan and I decided that we would move our routine non COVID-19 care patients from Manhattan to our nearby Bronx facility. The Bronx VAMC is also very capable and well-staffed. Both of these outstanding medical centers provided experienced and skilled staff and were very well-led across their senior management teams. We all felt comfortable with this decision and instituted plans for patient movement to and from each medical center as we prepared to operationalize the decision and thus establish a COVID-19 positive and COVID-19 negative hospital to serve the Veterans and the civilian community of NYC.

In retrospect, this decision was one of the most obviously wrong decisions I made during the initial phases of the pandemic.

About seventy-two hours following the implementation of these COVID-positive and negative hospitals, cases of COVID-19 began occurring in the Bronx (our COVID-negative) facility. And COVID-negative patients continued to arrive at the ER of the Manhattan facility. We quickly recognized that what seemed like a reasonable decision to segregate infected and uninfected patients by facility was not going to work. We failed because the virus, of course, had a say in this decision. We also failed because although patients knew that they were sick, they did not necessarily know that they had COVID-19. They, therefore, went to the health facility that they trusted with their care. Interrupting that trust was not going to be successful.

The point that I am trying to make here is that during a crisis, you as a leader do not have all the answers. Make a reasoned decision when you have a greater likelihood of success than failure, but recognize that all the information is not available, and waiting for all the information will potentially cost lives. When making these decisions, you must be humble enough to change course if your decision results in an unexpected or negative outcome. Do this decision-making and evaluation transparently, acknowledge your decision didn't work, and change course. Don't sugarcoat the outcome. The value to your workforce is that they will understand your ego will not get in the way of organizational success. I encourage the reader to spend some time looking at the interviews with leaders in post-crisis events. Decide if they are being brutally honest or trying to justify their poor decisions. Any statement that begins with "out of an abundance of caution" can be translated and interpreted clearly. By definition, a once-in-a-hundred-year event with rapidly evolving implications requires a leader move quickly to reposition their organizational capabilities for maximum impact. Own your decisions, review them continuously, and right the ship as quickly and transparently as possible. Your willingness to change direction when the results of a rapid decision become clear will foster significant agility in decision-making from other leaders across your organization.

During a crisis, leaders cannot wait for all the data to be analyzed in order to make a potential decision clear and low risk. Nor can they accumulate all the SMEs and second-order effect counsel that are usually present as a leader makes a deliberate decision regarding routine challenges. Those waiting for all the data and for consensus to be reached will find their organizations frozen in place, watching the evolving events of the crisis overwhelm them, while the chance for a decision and the opportunity to control their organization's future slip away. Remember, there are no silver bullets, and unlike in the drills, there is no "right" decision. When all your options are bad or have unknown effects, you can only trust your instincts and be ready to change course when the fog of war starts to lift.

We established the following principle for all VHA leaders and ourselves: Get to 60 percent on any decision. At 60 percent, the probability of success is greater than the probability of failure. Make your decision and then run with it. But always be humble enough, just as with the New York and Bronx hospital decision on COVID-19 positive and COVID-19 negative patient segregation, to actively observe the effects of your decision and change course if you need to. The Manhattan and Bronx decision were a perfect example of the 60-percent rule. We had enough information to make what I thought was an obvious and safe decision that quickly turned out to be wrong.

I still cringe as I'm writing this because it seems so clear what I should have done in hindsight. In government service, there is little tolerance for these changes in direction by the media. The media, for example will exploit these changes in direction supported by purported SMEs who will have significant commentary about what government leaders should have done, after the fact.

Joan, as the VISN leader, was an extraordinary partner in these events. She was experienced and imperturbable as we reexamined our decisions and processes and then corrected our way ahead. There was huge value in this recognition that we would have to operate facilities with COVID-19 negative and COVID-19 positive patients housed within the same building. Because of this new or amended decision to collocate patients, we discovered that there were ways to protect all our patients within our facilities from infection, and if we failed, we would not contain the infection as rapidly or as effectively as possible. Failure would create huge risk for patients and staff. The failure to recognize this fact in civilian and state-run (non VHA) nursing homes across the nation would cause the eventual infection and death of hundreds of patients.

It was at this point that we recognized that we must operate COVID-19 positive and COVID-19 negative *neighborhoods* in the same facility, even in our long-term care facilities. The key to safely delivering this decision was to ensure no individual broke the infection control protocols and move between COVID-19 positive and COVID-19 negative neighborhoods. As previously described, someone delivering trays of food from the facility kitchen could not go in and out of the COVID-19 positive areas of operation. We had to establish a transfer or exchange point for all materials and personnel types in a hospital in order to protect against the transfer of the virus. As such, we reexamined every one of the hundreds of processes across the hospital (and nursing home) and restaffed every single one that required movement into and out of COVID-19 areas in order to ensure patient and employee safety. Our next challenge was to ensure transparency of these decisions, propagate the dissemination of lessons learned across our entire nationwide network, and enable the VHA to operate as the agile learning organization we aspired to be.

These decisions impacted the consumption rate of materials already in short supply. I will discuss the logistics system later, but the impact on critically short supplies was difficult to quantify as we were breaking well-understood processes and quickly implementing new complex processes for even what seemed to be simple tasks. For example, most blood specimen analysis is centralized, and specimens are transported by semiautomated vacuum "tube" systems to the central lab. The protection of receiving lab personnel when opening the specimen containers had to be trained and reviewed. The presence of a phlebotomist to draw the blood specimen required a specialized employee to remain in the COVID-19 positive neighborhood for their entire shift. It also required additional personnel competent in blood specimen retrieval from patients to cover COVID-19 negative neighborhoods. The complex staffing and material consumption rates challenged our decision support and staffing matrix tools with every process we transformed.

I want to note that we were asking for a huge amount of flexibility and resiliency from many types of staff members in implementing changes like this. Our food service teams, environmental management staff, administrative assistants, IT teams, engineers, and many more were not typically trained in things like infection control. Most had never worn an N95 mask, not to mention a full gown, shield, and respirator. When people look back at the COVID-19 pandemic and recognize the "frontline" workers, they are obviously drawn to the clinical staffs, EMTs, and even their local grocery store workers who visibly went to work every day to fight this virus and keep our nation going. The men and women behind the scenes in these hospitals who fed our Veterans and staff, made the technology work, and made the wards clean and safe didn't sign up to go into these infected spaces when they took their jobs, but they did it anyway. They are among VHA's many unsung heroes.

CHAPTER EIGHT

Management By Directive and Regulation

VHA IS A HUGE organization. As of June 2022, more than 371,000 VHA employees are spread over fifty states, Puerto Rico, and multiple islands in the western Pacific Ocean to include the Philippines. This places VHA, with an annual budget approaching $100 billion dollars, within the top one hundred organizations in the nation from a revenue standpoint. For well over twenty years, VHA had grown into a top-down driven, overwhelmingly structured organization. Senior leadership usually exercised authority by the generation of written directives and regulations that are either published in the federal register or published and disseminated directly across thousands of operating sites. Literally hundreds of these regulations and directives are generated by the leadership team, "affectionately" referred to as "The Central Office" each year. The central office is physically located across Pennsylvania Avenue from the White House and is housed in an ancient GSA-owned building that rises ten stories above street level.

The myriad of directives and regulations are sometimes codified in the Federal Register, where any stakeholder (usually from outside the VHA itself) can comment in writing during their formulation, and the VHA is required to respond (also in writing) to all input. This process can take many months and results in complex and disjointed documents that are confusing and difficult for VISN and medical center directors to understand, let alone implement. This slow process is poorly designed to respond to rapidly evolving challenges. Somehow this process as described is supposed to deliver a transparent and responsive health system to all stakeholders. It delivers quite literally the opposite, in my opinion. A robust labor force assigned to this directive and regulation-generating work generates these documents, asks for input, attempts to reach consensus from stakeholders within and outside the system, and then, if/when complete, directions for the operating units are published and attempts to implement the directive begin. To institute any substantive operational change can take years. This results in a painfully slow process for any attempt at transformation. The Government Accountability Office and numerous inspectors general have commented for years about this painfully slow and seemingly unresponsive process. Changing this painful system of decision-making was absolutely necessary.

Soon after I arrived at VHA in July 2018, I received a summary of some recently completed medical research that had been conducted at nine VHA medical centers. The study focused on those Veterans who had survived a suicide attempt, had been cared for in a VHA emergency room, and were being considered for discharge following their stabilization. Each surviving Veteran would receive follow-up care in an outpatient care setting after their discharge. This post discharge time period is recognized as an extremely high-risk time for any suicide attempt survivor. Additional suicide attempts or actual death from self-harm is dramatically higher in the weeks following discharge from a previous attempt. In the research study, each

Veteran, prior to discharge from the ER, was engaged by their ER provider with a signed "contract" that outlined follow-up care and communication requirements. Most importantly, the patient and the provider pledged, by their signature, that there would be daily telephonic contact between providers and the Veteran until the Veteran was safely transitioned to, and confident in, the care from their outpatient provider. The results of this research, conducted at nine VHA medical center ERs, indicated that future suicide attempts in those Veterans with these "contracts" were reduced by as much as 50 percent in the months following discharge from the ER. I was amazed at this level of success.

The following morning during my weekly leadership team meeting that included about fifty key organizational leaders from the central office in Washington, DC, I asked who was aware of the recently completed research. Other than the head of suicide prevention and the head of ER operations, no one. I verbally reviewed the results and presented the leadership team the following question, "What shall we do now?"

After a long and painful period of silence, the team began making suggestions that included the need to confirm the findings with additional studies. "How long will that take?" I asked. The answer? About two years. I was heartbroken.

Suicide is one of the most difficult and tragic causes of death we as individuals, medical professionals, families, and as a society encounter. There are no Americans who haven't been exposed to the "twenty a day" numbers of Veteran suicide. But here we were, in a perfect example of our lack of agility, with research results showing significant value in reducing future Veteran risk. This was not a high-risk intervention requiring new medications that might have some unknown patient risk.

It was solely a behavior-based intervention and commitment of the patient and provider to talk each day. "What was the downside risk?" I asked. "Well," they responded, "it might not work when we roll it out over the entire system." I believed it was worth the risk, as did the study investigators, the heads of emergency medicine, and suicide prevention.

We decided that morning to institute these Veteran survivor and provider contracts across the nation in every VHA ER within ninety days; no directives and no regulations. The head of Emergency Medicine would generate a simple email to all ER directors, and we would begin.

Skeptics unfamiliar with rapid decision-making were plentiful. However, within thirty days of the decision, we began receiving anecdotal reports of lives saved from around the country, including a Veteran in New York who stood on the railing of a bridge, and before he jumped to his certain death, he placed his right hand over his heart. His hand touched his printed "contract" in his shirt pocket. Startled, he stepped down off the edge of the railing, back onto the sidewalk of the bridge, and pulled out the contract. He reread it and called his provider (while standing on the bridge), whose personal cell number was on the contract, and said, "OK, you saved me; please come get me!" We received multiple reports like this. A second Veteran in North Carolina called his family from his cell phone and said goodbye to them. He then removed the battery from his phone so he couldn't be traced. His family knew he had a contract. They frantically called the VA Medical Center and were connected to the provider whose name was on the Veteran's contract. This was the same provider he had met during the ER visit that occurred following his previous suicide attempt. In the preparation of his contract, the Veteran had revealed the location he would go to in order to commit a future act of self-harm. Local police were dispatched to that location, an enclosed garage, and found the Veteran inside a vehicle with the engine running. He was rescued alive and brought to the VAMC for further inpatient care.

The widespread organizational pride in this rapid rollout and its anecdotal effect was amazing. Not only did this decision save lives, but it also demonstrated the validity of rapid decision-making and began to show the employees and the leaders of the VHA that they could transform themselves with a level of rapidity and agility none had thought was possible.

Later in the same week, as the suicide study was published, I conducted what I called "mail call." This meeting consisted of a very small group of central office leaders to include the acting under secretary (me), the chief of staff, and my executive assistant. We met every few days in my office to review communications and invitations for speaking engagements. We also reviewed documents requiring my signature. One of the documents we reviewed that week for signature was a request from a medical center director to change the name of the street her medical center was located on from "Street" to "Avenue." I had no idea at the time why this was important, but it was important enough for a senior leader in charge of a medical center to send the document forward.

The original request document now enclosed in a two-inch-thick binder of concurrence documents that dated back up to two years. It had required more than twenty offices to review the request and obtain signatures from each of those office leaders. When one of those reviewers had a question, it was rerouted back to the requesting medical center, and the concurrence process was restarted. This was a perfect example of what needed to be changed in how we ran this organization—two years of a document moving from one layer of the organization to another that had *nothing* to do with how we provided care for Veterans. There was no visibility to the requesting medical center director of where the decision request was in the system except that it was "in concurrence."

Decisions in any organization, no matter the size, should always be made by the first-line leader who has all the information to make the decision and understand the consequences. I used this specific request as an example of what needed to change to transform the VHA into an agile organization. Consider how demoralizing it is for a medical center director with a staff of more than 2000 employees and a budget in the hundreds of millions of dollars to relegate this level of decision-making to a poorly responsive central office. I found this model of decision-making infuriating, demeaning, and disrespectful of the regional and local leaders we had entrusted to run our care delivery system. Worse, it was a waste of time when Veterans were relying on us.

In every leadership decision, there is the risk of failure. Intolerance of even minor failure by oversight committees and the media is perpetuated by organizations like GAO and the OIG who write reports months or years after a decision is made and implemented and the outcome is realized. This results in an extraordinarily long backlash to an outcome that may have been corrected long before the GAO/IG report is even generated. I am not arguing that OIG and GAO have no value. But when their reports are often generated with such a significant delay, they have the unintended effect of reducing the willingness of current leaders to make decisions. Or those leaders will "turf" all decisions to higher levels of leadership, making experienced professionals into little more than middle managers on a concurrence sheet.

As I approached an attempt at correcting this issue, I wanted VHA leaders at all levels to learn from decisions that did not have the desired outcome as quickly as possible. I also wanted decision-making to not be dependent on me reading a research summary. I described this as making the office of the under secretary superfluous to decision-making except in those rare cases that impacted budget, very high-level strategy, or executive branch policy. I presented this thought to our monthly VISN leader meeting. There was significant skepticism that I was serious. Implementation of this delegation of decision authority would restore operational decision-making authority to the leaders we had placed around the country. This was a departure from decades of decision-making authority being centralized in Washington, DC, removing most authority from leaders managing multibillion dollar regional health care systems. I presented my opinion that this system was disrespectful toward each one of them as they spent months or years waiting to get a decision that added no value, and support for this delegation of authority arose in the regional leaders.

In order to facilitate organizational and individual leader learning, every individual with a stake in the outcome of a decision must be present for and participate in a decision. I ask you to think back to the inflatable "golf dome" story from Afghanistan in 2003, where every operational leader participated every twelve hours with every other leader and the commanding general. Only with this model can a senior leader develop and promote shared accountability and shared decision-making that ensures rapid, agile, and informed decisions. This previous statement is only true if the senior leader encourages and welcomes input and challenges. This can, at times, be uncomfortable and even messy. But it rapidly reveals consensus or if, in fact, there is none. An example of this occurred in the suicide prevention contract I discussed previously. The manner in which that decision was made failed to recognize the role of the local ER leaders in this decision. As the director of VHA emergency services called them all together in a video conference, there was substantial resistance based upon valid workload and staffing concerns. We could have moved that implementation even faster if we had acknowledged a key stakeholder's absence when I made that decision or if I had allowed the ER program director to discuss the impending decision before the email that rapidly implemented the new process.

In 2016, I was serving as the principal deputy under secretary for health at VHA and recognized the same problems that I have just discussed. I introduced the concept of a command or operations center like I saw in Afghanistan and elsewhere in the military. The purpose of the operations center would be to ensure that every decision at any level would become transparent across the organization at all levels. The head of operations at that time worked operational updates by conference calls and monthly meetings in which the VISN leaders would fly into Washington, DC, or join a conference call and discuss problems. Agendas were filled, for the most part, with central office updates and decisions, and the VISN leaders sat quietly giving occasional input. This concept of an operations center was foreign to the then chief of operations, and his response was courteous but ambivalent.

I approached the then under secretary for health, Dr. David Shulkin. David was intrigued but noncommittal. He did, however, allow me to establish an operations office in vacant space on the tenth floor of the VA headquarters to test the concept. In 2016, we established an operations center and installed significant video and audio technology in an office that would accommodate about twenty-five personnel. The 2016 hurricane season that followed was the first significant hurricane season since 2012. There were fifteen named storms with seven hurricanes and four major hurricanes from June to November. Through the use of this temporary operations center, we successfully supported multiple hurricane response events with primary staffing provided by our office of emergency management team relocated from West Virginia.

We responded to the first hurricane to hit Florida since 2005, Hurricane Hermine, in 2016, caused extensive coastal flooding, resulting in five fatalities and five hundred million dollars in property damage. The VHA deployed support for displaced Veterans and supported affected areas with mobile pharmacies, feeding, and even mobile treatment centers. The most significant storm of the season was Hurricane Matthew. Matthew was a monster category 5 storm that devastated Haiti and moved up the east coast of Florida and the coasts of Georgia and South and North Carolina, causing significant coastal flooding, killing forty Americans, and causing billions of dollars in damage. For the VHA, the ability to manage a multistate response to include actual evacuation of our Charleston, Virginia, hospital would not have been possible without the visibility provided by the operations center. The Ralph Johnson VHA medical center is a 149-bed facility located on a near sea level peninsula with multiple other civilian hospitals in Charleston. This area is historically flood-prone, and the storm surge from Matthew was predicted to be ten to twenty feet in height.

Protecting vulnerable patients and ensuring their safety required moving them out of the potential path of the storm. This required the integration of wheeled ambulances and high clearance mobility vehicles, along with complex coordination between nurse and provider delivery teams at both Charleston and receiving VHA hospitals. Adequate medications, oxygen, IV fluids, and staff to accompany patients were just a few of the challenges completed in preparation for a storm that would cause nearly sixteen billion dollars in damage to the United States. The Charleston Medical Center supports over 65,000 Veterans in South Carolina and the adjacent states. As part of this supported population, there were more than three hundred spinal cord-injured Veteran patients located across the Charleston community. All of them needed to be contacted and their safety assured by family members or to be moved into a secure VHA medical center out of harm's way.

Without the operations center, the medical center director and their staff would be alone in responding and coordinating. We quickly learned that we could substantially unload the local leadership and staff by coordinating and supporting their decisions. As the storm progressed and the hospital was emptied, the facility needed to remain available for Veterans and community members who had refused to evacuate. The leadership team moved into the facility and remained in contact with the operations center throughout the storm's landfall. The ability of every VHA leader across the nation to hear (in real time) the challenges that the Charleston medical center director was facing, and the emotion of impending loss was an extraordinary learning experience for every leader across VHA.

Another important lesson in this model of leadership is that this type of visibility is not an excuse for a leader in a faraway central office to assume control of decision-making from the leader actually on the ground. Decisions, such as an evacuation, should be made by those closest to the impending risk. That decision-making delegation is difficult for strong decision-oriented senior leaders to implement. There is substantial value to helping frontline, on-the-ground leaders be able to "see" the entire region and its capabilities as well as potential decision risks. But these complex decisions must be made locally. The role of the national operations center was to support and facilitate and make sure the implementation of the decision by the medical center leader is executed with the greatest chance of success. That week, the Charleston VHA medical center evacuated but did not close. Over one hundred employees remained in the facility through the storm that inundated Charleston and flooded the hospital grounds. They continuously supported the Veteran community and its most vulnerable patients, even when the facility was surrounded by multiple feet of sea water.

It was my impression that the 2016 hurricane season, and most significantly, the response to Hurricane Matthew, validated for VA leaders the value of a national health operations center. When I left VHA in early 2017, as Dr. Shulkin moved from under secretary to become secretary of the VA, the VHA health operations center was, unfortunately, shut down and abandoned. Its personnel were repurposed, but the equipment allowing nationwide communication was left in place, and VHA returned to the use of desk phones and conference calls to manage all emergency events, even those involving widespread natural disasters.

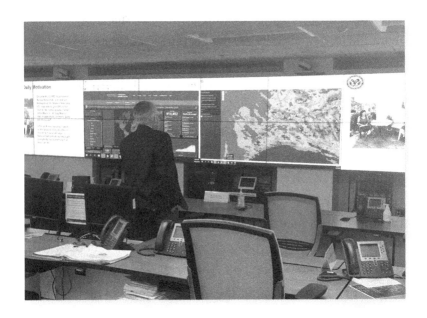

P4: Health operations center VHA

This rapid return to previous work processes demonstrates an important lesson for all leaders: **Sustained transformational change requires followership for an idea, not the popularity of a person in positions of leadership.** Many inside VHA followed me because I was respectful and courteous to them. What the organization really needed was a sense of ownership of this new transformative operating idea by enough of the VHA leaders so that it could be sustained. I did not deliver that sense of organizational ownership when I departed in early 2017 despite our 2016 Hurricane Matthew success. Emergency management personnel understood shared decision-making and the role of an operations center and welcomed the tool. Senior leaders above them did not feel a sense of ownership necessary for long-term sustainment and, therefore, the tipping point of engagement to sustain this new capability did not exist.

Many decades ago, a major survey company conducted an employee survey that revealed that in any organization, the tipping point for sustainability of transformation was about 25 percent. This meant that, in order to make change in any organization, about 25 percent of employees need to share a leader's vision for the future. In addition, 65 percent of employees are good citizens and will follow the 25 percent . There are about 10 percent of employees in any organization that are, frankly, on the wrong bus.[28] Your job as a leader is to always seek to find the 25 percent who share your vision. Many new leaders think their job is to take on the 10 percent who will actively work against you. That, in my opinion, is the job of human resources leaders. That 10 percent will use up all your time and energy should you choose to engage them. By engaging that 10 percent, you will find yourself in a morass of human resource-related processes, and your time and energy to actually lead the organization will be gone.

I have applied the "find the 25 percent" rule every day and in every situation for more than thirty years. I am looking for the two to three out of ten in a room that share my vision for the future or whatever I am engaged in with the group. Think about your last meeting when someone was obviously disengaged. You could tell by their body language that they were having no part in whatever you were talking about. Most of us move our attention to that person because we believe we just need to convince them that what we are saying is right or we have the right action to take. **What I am trying to say is that your attention as the visionary leader should be on those who are already on board with you. It should focus on the 25 percent and to**

identify and provide tools for success to those who share your vision and will implement change in the direction you seek, even if you are not present. Those are the individuals who will deliver lasting change, and that is what I failed to deliver as the principal deputy under secretary for health in 2016 and early 2017 at VHA. I failed to deliver the 25 percent-tipping point for transformative change that would sustain the organization toward the vision I had articulated and demonstrated.

In June 2018, just prior to my return to the VHA, Congress passed a complex law entitled the MISSION (Maintaining Internal Systems and Strengthening Integrated Outside Networks) Act that, among other things, transformed the way VHA purchased care in the community. The MISSION Act sought to correct many of the problems that occurred following the implementation of legislation that was passed following the 2014 access to care crisis in Phoenix, Arizona. That legislation implemented a program entitled "Choice." The 2014 legislation improved the ability for Veterans to choose community-provided care if VHA was unable to provide care that was reasonably accessible from a time or distance standpoint. The law sought to abolish the need for waiting lists and delays in care. The MISSION Act further refined this purchase of care by requiring the VA secretary to implement nationwide guidance on access standards for Veterans. These included standards on acceptable drive time and the number of days until available appointments that, if exceeded, would trigger the need for VHA to offer Veteran's care, delivered in their community health care systems (outside VHA). This legislation was contested by those who believed it could be used to "privatize" the VHA and move all Veteran care into the community. It was my impression that this legislation required absolute transparency on the part of

VHA, and the provisions of the law must be implemented uniformly across the thousands of VHA treatment sites. This was going to be a very tall order. Only using a capability like the operations center could we manage the uniform rollout of the MISSION Act and demonstrate the value of rapid learning that could occur in a venue such as this.

The ability to demonstrate transparency to all leaders, oversight organizations, Veteran Service Organizations, and, most importantly, to the leaders and employees of the VHA could only be delivered through the transparency and expertise of the health operations center, which is why, shortly after my arrival at VHA as the executive in charge, reinstated the health operations center in the fall of 2018. As part of the implementation of the new MISSION Act law, VA developed and delivered a simplified software tool that allowed providers the ability to communicate to Veterans when they were eligible for care in the community. That "Decision Support Tool" would quickly become essential to our success and a focus for media, the White House, and congressional attention.

The development of this tool was under the direction of the Assistant Under Secretary for Health for Community Care Kameron Matthews, MD. Kameron is a graduate of Johns Hopkins School of Medicine and received a Juris Doctor degree from the University of Chicago School of Law. She was serving as the senior leader whose primary responsibility was to develop the commercial delivery network that would institute the purchase of commercial care under the MISSON Act. Her success led her to become the chief medical officer of the VHA in 2020. Kam is an extraordinary talent who understood this complex law and quickly built a delivery team of experts to implement the required systems and processes included in the provisions of the law on time and successfully. Most importantly, she created performance standards that required concurrence from leaders throughout the VHA, the VA secretary, Veteran advocacy groups and congressional oversight committees. She would adeptly garner the support of these stakeholders without exception. Finally, she empowered the team that would design and implement the Decision Support Tool essential to this work.

The actual fielding of a homegrown software system in VHA is handled by a sister organization in the VA named the Office of Information Technology (OIT). At that time, OIT was led by Jim Gfrerer. Jim served in the Marine Corps for twenty-eight years and retired at the rank of colonel, deploying to four combat tours in the process. Jim delivered a sense of duty, experience, and partnership to the MISSION Act implementation that was, in my view, both welcome and essential.

We brought Jim and the OIT team into our daily health operations center briefings to ensure a seamless fielding of the new software capability and transparency to OIT of any frontline problems we faced. We also would need stability of the software platform at scale. The VHA performs about 250,000 provider-based patient encounters daily, so the ability of a software system to remain stable at this level of use across the entire nation was a massive undertaking that would only be successful if OIT leadership and VHA were completely aligned. We physically demonstrated our partnership by having Jim and I sit side by side in the front row of the operations center meetings and each of us facilitating our teams' interactions, which were respectful and focused on problem-solving in a transparent manner.

Jim's team delivered flawlessly, but we also needed to provide online training to this new software system and track training completion rates for over 200,000 employees. The tools we developed to track training success were displayed daily across the eighteen VISNs and 175 medical centers, showing which VISN and medical center had finished training and where training acceptance was lagging. We could also see immediately the satisfaction of trainees with the provided product and correct or modify the training product while in use. All of this was facilitated by the transparency of a well-functioning operations center. These sessions also revealed a highly competitive regional leadership cadre across the system. When we openly posted performance rates in live video sessions of their peers, lagging performance was corrected without my intervention. These were both proud and extremely competent leaders across the system. All they needed was the data in order to perform and, just as importantly, an environment of mutual respect and support.

At times, there were difficult performance questions. I would highlight a high-performing region and then turn the group's attention to a lower-performing region with the following question, "VISN XX, help us understand why your performance is unique and what support you need to reach the success of the high-performing VISNs?" No leader wants that kind of attention. There are situations, however, where a leader needed significant help. What I was impressed with was the willingness of other regional leaders to support their fellow leader's success. This resulted in rapid organizational performance improvement without the influence of the central office or the office of the under secretary.

There is significant discussion in technical forums about how to handle data for a large organization. I am by no means a technical or data expert, but I need data quickly to manage an organization. VHA had developed and evolved a data platform that, in 2012, was placed into a performance platform called Strategic Analytics for Improvement and Learning (SAIL). It compiled data from twenty-seven different quality measurements and patient satisfaction levels and then compared performance at different VHA medical centers across the enterprise. SAIL was overlayed with a rating system that publicly assigned "stars" to medical center performance on a scale of one to five.

The weighting of these performance metrics was not sufficiently transparent and was conducted by a team of well-intentioned data specialists within VHA. This rating system resulted in a poorly understood system that, on a quarterly basis, publicly released VHA hospital ratings and, in response, required lower-performing hospitals to create corrective action plans. Because of the complexity of the metrics, the team from SAIL found it necessary to perform assistance visits to help local leaders understand their data. I found that this system was well-intentioned, but the application of "stars" was not significantly helpful. It created an adversarial relationship between the data managers and the medical center director responsible to chart the course for local organizational performance. It also made Veterans believe that their local hospital, who perhaps had received one or two stars, was a bad hospital, which was almost never the case. Because these ratings were comparing facilities within the enterprise, the lowest-performing hospitals could still be better than their local non-VHA community facilities or even the best in their city, but there was no way to compare them. These reports fed the media's appetite for scandal within VHA under the auspices of "transparency" that often had little to do with the care being provided but was intensely damaging to both our facilities and providers' credibility in a community.

I believe that performance "data" is always a corporate asset. It should not be owned, managed, manipulated, or released by a single office in an organization. It should be accumulated in a readily accessible location and available to any leader who needs data to make a decision. It is acceptable to provide analysts and talent that will help the local leader manipulate and portray the data effectively, but it should never be used as a performance weapon. We had come very close to using data as a weapon and, therefore, we envisioned the standup of the operations center as the single point of definitive organizational data. Any disagreements on the validity of data would be resolved by the operations center data leads. We found that in response to SAIL, many local leaders had developed their own data-gathering systems to identify any problems and correct those problems before the SAIL star ratings were released because their reputations were on the line. Those local systems' data often conflicted with SAIL, and we established a mechanism for the resolution of conflicting data without a broad statement of change in data use policy, thus promoting transparency and transparent decision-making on performance improvement.

On the day the MISSION Act mandated that the new community care system go live, during June 2019, I spent the day in Montana with the Senate Veterans Affairs Committee ranking member (now Chairman) Senator Jon Tester. We toured care delivery sites in his state, and he and I participated virtually in a nationwide health operations center briefing. We called from a VHA videoconferencing location from the Fort Harrison

VAMC in Helena, Montana. The rollout had gone smoothly across the nation, we had corrected performance problems immediately, and it appeared as we entered the nationwide performance update that we had delivered a resounding success. This success was demonstrated by the stability of the newly fielded software platforms as well as the training and acceptance of the new program by end users who were caring for Veterans every day. This was also a reflection of Kam Matthews' diligence in engaging system frontline leaders in the development of these performance tools.

The transparency we demonstrated to Senator Tester was a high-profile example of what we intended to deliver to every Veteran who chose us for their care. During the one-hour meeting, the operations center coordinated and hosted video sessions with every VISN leader across the nation who were able to present their problems and obtain resolutions or decisions while we were still on the call. In addition, problems that had been overcome using local innovation in one area and still existed in another were resolved by VISN leaders helping each other. They were learning from each other and reducing the need to send problems up the chain of command. I was extraordinarily proud of Kam, the people of VHA, and our IT colleagues who worked shoulder to shoulder with us to field a complex health delivery system under this new law. I thought that the MISSION Act, by its sheer complexity, was the greatest challenge our operations center would face outside of combat. COVID-19, however, would far exceed anything I could have ever imagined, but having a well-functioning and established operations center in place helped prepare us for what would come a few months later.

Bringing the operations center back to life was led by a robust team of operational, clinical, and administrative staff, with oversight counsel from the then Deputy VHA Chief of Staff Jon Jensen. Jon is an extraordinary and rare talent. A senior Army non-commissioned officer with combat experience, his love of Veterans and the employees of VHA is unmatched. Jon served in combat in Iraq and approached the VHA as he did any of his uniformed assignments. He expected performance excellence and would be right beside you to help deliver it anytime, day or night. Jon understood the concept of an operations center and was experienced in their performance and function. He had experienced this capability in combat and immediately saw its value. Jon ensured the team had everything they needed as we built, staffed, trained, and then tested the operations center and its ability to be accessed from VHA leaders at all levels and in all locations. He and the staff demonstrated the 25-percent rule. Find those who share your vision and let them bring it to life.

Jon soon moved to the position of chief of staff. In this position, Jon also had a broader responsibility. When I arrived at the VHA in 2016 as the principal deputy under secretary, our senior leader talent pool was almost nonexistent. The 2014 access crisis and unrelenting media attacks had decimated our senior leader ranks due to resignations, retirements, or transfers to other agencies. Our ability to recruit new talent was hampered by a culture based on punitive responses to unintended outcomes and years of negative media coverage. Reports from the GAO and OIG were delivered months or years after events had occurred; their reports were flaunted in the media, often providing little additional value as external analysis of problems. Regardless of their intent, the response was an attrition of leadership talent. In addition, those developing leaders who served one or two levels below a medical center director were often unwilling to accept a more senior leadership promotion because they feared the potential implication of a performance error on their future careers. Our ability to have a robust talent pool of applicants for medical center and VISN leadership positions was almost completely destroyed by years of punitive actions and salacious attacks. We had to rebuild our talent pool while working to improve our relationship with the oversight teams from the GAO and OIG. I hoped that we would increase the value of the work done by GAO and OIG while also enhancing the willingness of developing leaders to serve at the highest level of the organization.

In 2016, the annual survey of employee opinion of "Best Places to Work" in the federal government rated the Department of Veterans Affairs as sixteenth out of seventeen large federal agencies. I am proud to say that by 2022, that number would rise to five out of seventeen rated agencies, an extraordinary turnaround that is a testament to an extraordinary team that focused on taking care of its employees, even in the midst of a pandemic.

—

While serving as the Combined Joint Task Force (CJTF) 180 senior medical officer in Afghanistan, I had the honor of serving with a dynamic young one-star general by the name of Lloyd Austin. I served as his command surgeon and was dual assigned as the commander of the multinational medical task force. Then Brigadier General Austin has since gone on to serve at both the four-star level and is currently at the Pentagon as the secretary of defense. He is an extraordinary combat leader who taught many leadership lessons to those of us who served beside him. **One of the most important was to never enter combat with one of anything. The result would be a single point of failure. This tenant was part of our planning for combat casualty care and has stayed with me as a basic foundational principle of crisis response.** Years later, we needed to apply this principle to our VHA leadership team as quickly as possible. We were barely one deep in almost every position, and in most of those, the incumbent had been placed there as a temporary or time-limited assignment. Many others were retirement-eligible and weren't shy to tell you about it.

We began recruiting in earnest, and each of us on the leadership team sought talented candidates to interview and potentially join us. The Chief (as we called Jon Jensen) was essential to closing the employment contract with multiple potential candidates. Because our federal government pay scale for medical leaders was often substantially less than the civilian health sector, we usually attracted candidates who were former military or senior civilian health leaders coming to VHA in a desire to be part of the mission to care for America's heroes. Few were looking to start a career with us. Most just wanted to serve. It was an easy sell for the mission but much more difficult as we discussed the toxic and punitive culture that we promised was being transformed.

Jon articulated this better than anyone, and his credentials as a combat Veteran and reputation as an honest speaker had huge value. The Chief delivered two other areas of strong characteristics as we built the team that would engage COVID-19: First, he understood the need to balance external hires with promotion from within the ranks. That balance often eludes leaders trying to bring talent into an organization. Rising and talented internally promoted leaders will not stay with an organization if they do not believe their service is valued. That value is expressed in promotions and recognition. If every new leader is hired from the outside, and there is no chance for internal upward mobility, internal talent will eventually leave. We established an unwritten goal of one-third external hires and two-thirds promoted from within. That goal was difficult to achieve as many of the internal talented candidates were reluctant to accept highly visible (and, therefore, vulnerable) leadership positions until they were convinced that the culture of retribution was changing. Understanding the internal promotion and external hire balance ensured the preservation of extensive organizational knowledge and fostered trust in those working in the field. It also ensured that organizational diversity and experience would be promoted with newly hired external experienced leaders with diverse perspectives.

Second, Jon understood that this type of organizational transformation and rapid assimilation of new leaders required consistent and effective communication. Jon and a team of crisis communicators from Deloitte encouraged me to begin recording daily videos directed to all VHA employees. They adeptly recognized that during a crisis, all employees needed transparency and to hear from their leadership as much and as frequently as possible in a consistent way. In the absence of that level of communication, rumors and fear take over your organization. Trust in leadership communication only has value if it is followed by leadership action that aligns to the message being given. We have experienced this erosion of trust during the pandemic by the never-ending litany of local and national leaders who mandated mask usage and then were revealed as not complying with their own mandates. The erosion of trust in those leaders was significant and irredeemable. Employees will only follow a leader whose words are aligned to their own actions.

Early in my leadership career, I worked at a Midwest health care system that took great pride in their motto, "Our most important asset is our people." Like all slogans, those words needed to be confirmed by leadership action, or they were meaningless. During this time, the hospital I was working in was led by a dynamic and popular leader who served as the CEO. She articulated the motto regarding our people in almost every public and employee-facing speech.

During my tenure, there was a nurse, who will be named Sarah for the purposes of this book, serving on one of the nursing units. Sarah was a long experienced bedside care nurse and was recognizable as the only nurse employed by the system who still wore her nursing school cap. This unique headwear dates back to the beginning of the nursing profession and has been abandoned by most currently practicing nursing professionals. I always knew when Sarah was working when I walked onto her ward because, in addition to her medical talents, she was a nationally-recognized championship whistler. Her ability to whistle beautiful melodies was calming to her patients and all of us around her. Unfortunately, Sarah sustained a series of aging and bedside care delivery-related health challenges, and her four decades of service were coming to an end. Sarah loved nursing and tried to return to work despite significant physical challenges. She often said that we, her fellow employees, and patients, were her family.

Human resources eventually got involved and decided that this four-decade employee was no longer physically able to complete the tasks of bedside nursing, which is widely acknowledged as a physically demanding profession.

The story really begins here.

Instead of the health system leadership working to provide a respectful transition for Sarah and recognizing her decades of service to the system and the community, they terminated her.

Sarah received notice of her termination while working her shift when a senior HR administrator and two uniformed security officers arrived on the medical unit presented the document outlining her immediate termination based on her inability to provide "safe" care. Sarah was speechless. She could not grasp what was happening, nor could her colleagues. The HR administrator soon left the nursing unit after presenting the letter of termination, stating Sarah would get her final check in the mail. Sarah was then escorted out of the building by security officers walking on either side of her to the front door of the hospital and told not to return. Her name badge and keys to the medicine room were taken, and she was left outside the door. The conclusion of forty-plus years of service to the same employer ended with her weeping uncontrollably in the driveway under the covered portico and then slowly walking to her car to weep again before she drove away alone.

A week later, the popular young medical center leader was addressing a large gathering of employees about a new benefit of employment being offered by the system. She used the well-worn statement, "You know, our people are our most important asset." She was then shocked when she was loudly and universally booed by the audience, and several employees stood up and walked out.

In fairness, the CEO did not know about the termination of one of her 2,400 employees, nor should she have. But her chance to recover was now, and she missed it. She needed to ask about the issue, recognize Sarah, acknowledge the error of how egregiously this was handled, and finally ensure that every HR leader knew this type of behavior was unacceptable and violated the organization's core values. When none of that happened, employee attrition over the next year doubled as employees sought employment in another system that they believed lived its stated values.

CHAPTER NINE

The Use of Video To Facilitate Learning and Leadership

JON AND THE DELOITTE crisis communication team were persistent in convincing me of the need to communicate widely to all VHA employees in order to ensure every employee at every level knew how we were progressing with the pandemic, what we expected of them, and that I and the entire leadership team were available and sought their input and suggestions. There was, justifiably, a lot of fear across the VHA enterprise and the nation, especially in the early phases of the pandemic when people were being sent home from work, kids were being sent home from school, and there was significant conflicting guidance and "facts" being distributed from many sources about the COVID-19 virus.

For full disclosure, I loathe seeing myself on TV or on video. Over the course of my career, I have had the opportunity to deliver congressional testimony and participate in dozens if not hundreds of interviews on video or voice-only media formats, and I never watch them. It's pulling teeth to get me to do any of it. I recognize that I am probably the most self-critical person of anyone in history, though that might be an overstatement (in all of history, there must be someone worse). Despite that shortcoming and with the stated fact that I would never watch myself in one of these videos, Jon encouraged me, and I agreed that we should begin daily video messages distributed to all our VHA employees.

This effort was supported by a remarkable team of communications subject matter experts from Deloitte, led by Rosemary (Ro) Williams. Ro was a former assistant secretary of Public and Intergovernmental Affairs at the VA as well as the former deputy assistant secretary of defense for Military Community and Family Policy and had earlier in her career served for more than eleven years as senior and then executive producer for NBC News. She is a proven communicator and trusted counsel. Her understanding of unique elements of crisis communication was extremely valuable throughout this period. Ro was always willing to take on a crisis and make our response better.

Rosemary was accompanied in this work by Brian Hawthorne. Brian was the former White House liaison at VA and an Army Reserve senior NCO with service in Iraq as a medic whose expertise was written communication and effective message delivery for senior leaders. At his core, Brian was an advocate for those who are currently serving or have served the nation in uniform. He was able to refine messages when I stumbled or was too emotionally connected to an issue to communicate clearly. The final member of the team was Kate Shepard. Kate is a mental health professional who had developed an extraordinary grasp of psychology, economics, business strategy, and anthropology. She had used these skills to take on some of the most complex mental health challenges facing clients during her career and brought both a calming bedside manner (mostly for me when I didn't want to talk about something) and a keen eye for effective empathetic messaging to the COVID-19 communications efforts. These three experts supported the VHA internal communications team in the development of communications products that delivered the transparent communications to Veterans and employees that we needed, tackling both my personal communications efforts as well as tough topics, such as mask and vaccine requirements, canceling of in-person family visitations to patients, and even the riots following George Floyd's death. Delivering this unique crisis communication expertise when a large government agency is significantly challenged was the perfect role for an industry partner such as Deloitte.

The videos were initially created because I was no longer able to regularly travel, a staple of my previous employee engagement efforts. We were initially trying to replicate what were called employee townhalls that I would host at the medical centers when I visited, but these daily videos soon took on a life of their own. The team had decided that my messages were believable only if I was speaking from the heart without teleprompter or even written notes. We decided that we would keep each video to under three minutes and release them so that they were available to be seen early in each workday by employees across the nation and were not hidden on an intranet site somewhere. We decided that they must be accessible on any device as long as the employee had a link. The team would propose topics and do some research, but usually, the videos were about whatever I was thinking about and often were highly personal and emotional. For the most part, they were recorded from cell phones on a tripod, as the professional studio facilities that we had at VA Central Office were closed early in the pandemic. We recorded these messages mostly in my office as my first task when arriving in my office in the morning. We would record from a medical center when I could travel, and sometimes we would feature other VHA leaders.

Early in the pandemic, my then eighteen-year-old son Danny developed severe COVID-19 pneumonia while visiting his grandfather in Florida. He, his twenty-year-old sister, Becca, and my wife, Jenni, remained in Florida for several weeks as Danny struggled to recover. He developed severe bilateral pneumonia, and I experienced the absolute helplessness of working in Washington, DC, and being unable to be with my family or see my son who was suffering. One morning, with some encouragement from Kate, I spoke about this feeling in a video to the VHA employees and was met with an unbelievable outpouring of support from our people across the nation. Employees related similar feelings of helplessness as they faced the massive weight of performing their jobs and caring for their families whose lives were just as disrupted and challenged.

Thousands of individual responses came to my email inbox over the course of nearly a year that we recorded these daily videos. I tried to acknowledge each with at least a thank you. I learned so much from the responses and began to realize that my connection to employees was dramatically enabled using this communication tool, creating a unique connection between me as the executive in charge of a ninety-billion-dollar organization and the (then) more than 360,000 frontline VHA employees. I encouraged feedback and started dialogues with many employees I never would have met or interacted with without this effort. Leadership in crisis can be lonely, but these conversations and notes reminded me each day that I was connected to my workforce, a vibrant and dedicated group fighting by my side across the country.

Sometimes the videos would quickly be seen by more than 40,000 of our employees. Many leaders began their morning leadership stand-up meetings by watching them as a team and discussing the issues we covered in the videos. Some pretty emotional responses came back in emails to me, including the loss of family members to COVID-19. By the time I left VHA in July 2021, we had recorded more than 250 of these short messages, and I remain amazed at their power. One of them highlighted the loss of my brother later in 2020 from an uncared-for health-related issue that I believed occurred because of his unwillingness to go to a hospital during the pandemic.

My emotional and painful grieving plea to our employees was to take care of themselves and don't delay their own care. We had worried that Veterans and employees would delay care and suffer advanced cancer or worsening comorbid conditions if we didn't encourage care. When I lost my own brother because of exactly this series of events, it painfully validated our concerns.

We began to realize that our employees in the most hard-hit areas of the nation where COVID-19 was the most prevalent were taking less sick and vacation time than historically normal levels. This seemed to confirm a commitment to their fellow workers and patients. We discussed as a leadership team and in a video to employees the interpersonal connection of military unit members and the extraordinary bond of commitment between service members that are tested in combat. We also strongly encouraged our teams to take the leave they had earned. In addition, VHA employee retirements during this time went down significantly. The commitment of VHA employees to stay the course voluntarily is one of the most remarkable untold stories in this pandemic. Around them in the civilian health care systems, salaries were skyrocketing, and yet these amazingly competent VHA employees stayed the course in support of the mission and showed an unwillingness to abandon their fellow employees or their mission to care for America's Veterans.

Creating trust and connection between leaders and front-line employees can be very difficult and seem insurmountable for any size organization. The videos exposed the common humanity and fear that every one of us were experiencing across America and within the VHA itself. That connection, identifying that no matter what the organizational challenge we were facing, all of us as individuals were experiencing the same problems together. Those shared experiences created a shared humanity that had significant value to cementing the commitment of the workforce to the VHA team and its leadership.

Over the course of these videos and on camera, I donated blood for a monumental effort called the Million Veterans Program, received my COVID-19 vaccine and administered the vaccine to my fellow employees at VACO, gave a tour of the healthcare operations center, spoke with the secretary of Veterans Affairs, celebrated National Nurses Day with our chief nurse Dr. Beth Taylor, visited a PPE distribution site with our head of support services Deb Kramer, gave out awards, cele-brated retirements, and spoke with medical center and VISN directors in the field when I could travel. Some were impromptu, some were planned ahead of time, but none were ever scripted. Not wanting to let the cadence falter when I finally took a week of leave six months into the pandemic response, the team worked with a group of different VHA leaders to film a video every day I was gone. I even filmed one myself from my living room when I was forced to quarantine following a potential exposure (with a little help from one of my grandchildren).

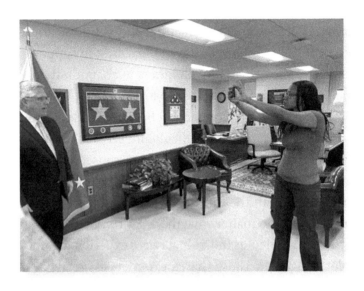

P5: Filming a daily video from my office in Washington, DC.

Some of the videos were recorded to dispel developing rumors. Early in the pandemic, many health care systems were experiencing a shortage of personal protective equipment. This was being reported daily by media across the nation. Pictures of health care workers in New York wearing plastic garbage bags spread across social media, and some VHA employees were rightfully concerned. I recorded a video and explained that VHA keeps operational stockage of these protective materials just like other health systems, but because of the nature of our nationwide emergency response mission, we keep an additional emergency storage supply. We believed early in the pandemic that we would be able to sustain our operations if our regular material suppliers continued to deliver materials as we ordered them. This, however, would change dramatically early in the pandemic, as I will discuss in detail.

Across VHA, we would never fall below fourteen days' supply in any single personal protective equipment (PPE) item. These items include various types of masks, gloves of different sizes, gowns, shoe coverings, and powered air purifying respirators (PAPRs) used in high-risk procedures, such as CPR and intubation of a patient who is unable to breath without mechanical support. By April 7th of 2020, we did experience some misdistribution of materials and, in response to the time it took to move materials around the nation, I instituted "emergency use" (crisis) orders to reduce rates of the consumption of these materials. This included a one-mask-per-day policy and one mask per week in lower-risk jobs. This lasted for nine days until the 16th of April, when we returned to "contingency" use authorities.

These policies were rightly controversial. Medical personnel in the United States are accustomed to disposing of materials after a single patient use and always having what they need to remain safe. The removal of that capability caused significant fear amongst our workforce who had never used protective equipment in more than one patient room. Throughout my career, it was considered an anathema to not change out of almost everything between patients, and I absolutely believe that we could have done better in the way we communicated those decisions. Our failure to do so effectively resulted in rumors of shortages that subsequent videos substantially helped to overcome.

As we moved through unprecedented demand for protective equipment, there were future scenarios that I could not predict how we would respond. When I didn't know the answer, I said "I don't know," but acknowledged the challenge anyway, and I promised that when I did know the answer, we would record it so employees could hear directly from me. This method of crisis communication promoted and created trust and ensured that every employee had the opportunity to hear directly from me without someone else interpreting my message. These videos flattened and shrank an extraordinarily large organization significantly, and many were forwarded outside the organization. Some turned into media/congressional inquiries, and I was proud to say that what I was telling our employees was exactly the same as what I would tell any reporter or member of Congress.

In addition to my video messages, the Chief began a monthly series of in-depth podcast-style interviews entitled *Chats with the Chief* that spent thirty to sixty minutes in-depth on individual subjects with leaders across the enterprise. They created the ability to go into great detail on any subject and highlight program leaders and medical center and VISN directors, who would share personal stories and talk about their own lessons learned and successes. With some encouragement and production direction from the Deloitte team, especially a young video producer and graphic designer named Peyton Marion, we discovered that Jon was a natural host, and each episode rapidly became very popular across the organization. They were directed at employees and worked to foster a deeper level of transparency that was not present previously. These podcasts were available publicly on various accessible sites. Employees told us they would often listen to them on their commutes home from work at the VHA.

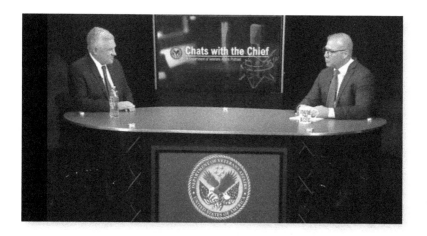

P6: Chats with the Chief. Jon Jensen and the author pictured

A final communications product that came out of the pandemic was called *COVID in 20,* (meaning in twenty minutes). The chief of emergency medicine started this program on his own (happily, without permission or support from central office) to spread emerging COVID-19 best medical practices across the ER services on a weekly basis and also meet the need for continuing education credits during a time when there were few opportunities for licensed practitioners to complete them. These episodes facilitated the standardization of rapidly changing medical processes and were fun, quirky, and incredibly effective. I called in several times to give updates, as did many other leaders, and through these tools, VHA was rapidly becoming one of the most effective medical learning organizations in the nation!

I cannot over emphasize the importance of regular and creative communications efforts for leaders, especially for those leading organizations through crises or disruptive transformation. Providing a consistent, accessible, and, if possible, two-way communications pattern gives employees a way to bring up issues internally instead of going to the media, Congress, or HR if they know they are going to be heard. Not all the feedback I received was positive by any means, and I was often shocked by what employees were willing to say to their leadership via email, but at least they were saying it to my face (so to speak). Over the years I was leading VHA during the pandemic, I would have email exchanges that spanned the emotional spectrum from sad, difficult, and angry to fun, celebratory, and gracious, and everything in between. I would receive advice, cooking recipes, requests for letters of recommendations, anniversary and birthday notifications, and much more, none of which would have likely been sent to me without my proactive communications pattern. Regardless, each of them was a personal conversation that I never would have been able to have on a typical site visit under a tight timeline, and I learned so much about the people that made up this incredible organization. I also quickly added our communications teams, at every level, to the list of unsung heroes of this pandemic response. I learned much about how difficult their jobs were, especially in communicating clearly and concisely about difficult, emotional topics that were likely to change and would almost certainly end up in a media or congressional inquiry. I probably wasn't their easiest or most willing spokesperson either, especially when it came to sharing my own feelings and struggles, but I certainly recognized the potential impact and was a fast convert.

CHAPTER TEN

Ensuring a Common Picture and Ensuring Diversity of Thought, Experience, and Ideas

BY EARLY FEBRUARY 2020, barely two months after my initial call with Paul Kim about this new disease, the rapidly expanding operational pace demanded that we ensure all leaders had a common operating picture of the challenges that faced us. McKinsey personnel had been briefing the most senior leadership of VHA and was accurately predicting two weeks in advance what American health care systems in specific regions might need to respond to. They were also presenting data on other countries and their national health systems pandemic response. I was convinced by all my previous experience that it was essential that every operational leader at every level heard and saw the same thing we in the senior leadership team were seeing. We began conducting a daily briefing from the operations center team and incorporated our McKinsey and Company partners into the briefing. McKinsey would present their view of the future, and the regional leaders at each of the eighteen VISNs would confirm or correct the McKinsey presentation. The VISN directors themselves would brief what they were seeing or contradict the model being presented in real time. This dynamic became a unique venue in the world to present a potential future model and then test its accuracy almost immediately with input from those delivering actual care in the communities being discussed.

We further created time for each VISN leader to discuss their challenges. This would include shortages of materials, consumable supplies, facility challenges, and real-time expanding patient volume. The ability to manage the flow of elective health care while at the same time responding to the potential of massive numbers of respiratory-compromised patients created immediate tension across the system. Our decision to delay non-emergent care for elective patients so that we could accept critically ill patients with COVID-19 created a tension grounded in the access standards we discussed previously for the MISSION Act. There was significant sensitivity that we could not reduce access to care, or we might find ourselves back in the 2014 access to care crisis. Therefore, the senior medical officers in each facility and every VISN began meeting with central office medical leaders (Kam Matthews and Chief Nursing Officer Beth Taylor) to ensure no emergent Veteran patient was delayed in their care.

Simultaneously, every commercial health system that operated near our VHA facilities was experiencing the same challenges. Each of those commercial delivery systems were delaying acceptance of elective cases and, therefore, community care-referred Veterans began to experience reduced community healthcare access as pandemic-caused hospitalizations increased throughout communities.

Every VISN completed a standardized operational PowerPoint slide each day, which was projected through the operations center to the entire VHA national delivery system. Verbal comments from the VISN leader were briefed "by exception." By this, I mean they briefed what was not already obvious on the slide or if there was something incorrect on the screen. They didn't enumerate what was going well. They spoke to risk and needed support. I ask the reader to remember the briefing model I introduced from Afghanistan earlier.

Each VISN took no more than two minutes so that all participants could hear from the entire nation in thirty-six minutes or less. With the other portions of the brief to include the McKinsey review of the civilian health care system challenges and the occupancy rates of civilian hospitals, we completed all of this in about an hour, starting at 7:45 EST every morning. We included a two-week prediction of what individual areas of the country would run out of ICU or medical beds in the next fourteen days. This allowed us to understand our own capability to potentially support civilian and potential non-Veteran health care needs well before the city, county, or region in peril even asked for support. This was briefed down to the county level across the entire nation by exception only. By this, I mean that we would discuss only those areas where it appeared beds of any type were going to be overwhelmed. This briefing model became very efficient. It took some time and a few nudges to those who wanted to brief on success, but with time, the entire team began to understand the value of this precious time. This time was essential to approach and solve problems. It was not unusual for a VISN not heavily engaged in the pandemic to respond with "nothing to report" and move immediately to the next VISN. I considered this extraordinary maturity on the part of those leaders.

As we continued through the pandemic, these briefings also became a way to track how quickly things could move. On March 9th, the New Orleans mayor reported the first case of

COVID-19 in the city of New Orleans. Within weeks, the entire city health care delivery system was at capacity and was at risk of running out of available beds. VISNs could see how one case in a neighboring VISN quickly became hundreds of lives at risk so they could prepare themselves and their teams.

The New Orleans VA Medical Center (NOVAMC) was a new facility built after Hurricane Katrina destroyed the prior VA medical center. The newly completed facility was designed to not only be hurricane proof but to also be infinitely configurable. This meant that we had the ability to modify an individual patient room up or down with the acuity needs of the patient. Individual room head walls (the head of the bed) were designed with the ability to convert a regular inpatient acute medical or surgical room into an ICU in a few hours. The ability to deliver centralized oxygen and complex monitoring was unique to this design. The VISN 16 Director Skye McDougall and the NOVAMC Director Fernando Rivera decided to convert the entire hospital into a one hundred bed-plus ICU after we had discussed the prediction of overwhelmed hospital beds for this community.

Fernando and Skye were incredibly experienced in emergency operations, and Fernando understood the facility he helped rebuild better than anyone, as he had led NOVAMC since 2015. The decision to increase critical care capacity by five times, however, would place increased staffing demand for critical care nurses upon the facility and its already stressed staff. During our daily national operations update, Skye requested personnel support in the form of critical care nurses, respiratory therapists, and laboratory personnel.

VISNs without a significant number of COVID-19 patients immediately (even during the HOC update) began promising personnel, and within a few hours, more than fifty critical care nurses and personnel with specifically requested skills were preparing to deploy to New Orleans. As the pandemic ravaged the community and the NOVAMC filled with patients, a further shortage of ventilators was also identified by NOVAMC leadership.

During the early phases of the pandemic, Governor Cuomo had requested thirty thousand ventilators for the state of New York. He had predicted his need for this number by April or May as the pandemic surged. A high-profile disagreement on the number of ventilators needed occurred between President Trump and the governor after a presidential press conference. (The reader should recall the hospital ship USNS Comfort that was delivered to New York Harbor and then released a few weeks later.) By the first week of April, downstate New York had 6500 ventilators in use on patients. Thousands of ventilators were delivered to New York in response to the governor's request. By April 15th, barely thirteen days later, the governor of New York announced in a press conference that he was redistributing ventilators to Michigan and Maryland because demand in New York had subsided. Movement of this complex equipment and its supporting materials is not simple to coordinate and execute. It is this political overlay that confounded supplies of essential materials across the nation. Health operations executives in both the civilian and federal sectors are highly adept at running complex health delivery operations. The involvement of politicians only complicated this response to possible patient need. There are no clearer lessons learned in this pandemic than the need for senior operational health delivery experts to manage the movement of materials and patients and personnel to support the American people in a nationwide crisis.

The ventilators' request by the VISN 16 leader occurred during our operations center call and was propagated in order to support the rapidly escalating mission of civilian and Veteran respiratory critical care by the VISN 16 leader. The VISN 23 director, Robert McDivitt, whose region of responsibility is the upper Midwest, immediately identified the ventilators needed, understood the dire and urgent request, and arranged trucking to have those lifesaving pieces of equipment transported and on the ground in New Orleans by the next morning. The key to this type of agility is transparent communication, trust, and shared learning. This also demonstrates the efficiency of solving problems rapidly at the lowest leadership level possible. This type of learning is enabled by trust between leaders that support received today will reverse direction at some point in the future. This rapid deployment of materiel is an example of the agility demonstrated in VHA and should be contrasted to decisions made by non-medical experts serving in elected leadership positions.

If this had been a wartime response where we were discussing the movement of ammunition supplies, the involvement of a president and governor in an open disagreement about the amount of ammunition that was needed and in what location would have been viewed as ludicrous. Medical operations experts across the nation viewed the early April exchange between the New York governor and the president of the United States in the same manner.

My overwhelming fear was that this model of "whack-a-mole" or flooding support wherever it was demanded could not be maintained and that COVID-19 would simultaneously infect the entire nation. I have discussed previously that the VHA hurricane, flood, or earthquake response contingency model was developed so that the entire VHA enterprise would align itself to support a single geographic region compromised by such an event. In this COVID-19 emerging pandemic, we redesigned that single regional response system to identify and plan for up to four areas of the nation under the most pressure for COVID-19 critical care admissions. We then regionally assigned the fourteen remaining VISNs to the role of operational reserve. These fourteen VISNs would provide support unless trends in case numbers or admissions to VHA or community hospitals suggested that increasing local demand required suspension of their support. In that case, their support would be replaced by another VISN. Trust between leaders was essential to maintaining this agile system of supported and supporting VISNs. In order to avoid duplication of effort, Renee Oshinski, as the chief of operations, divided the VISNs assigned to each of the anticipated challenged VISN in a three to four supporting to one supported VISN model. The trust between Renee and the VISN leaders was also essential in executing these assignments. We were asking leaders to voluntarily give up capacity or a capability in the middle of the crisis and trust that if COVID-19 would increase in their region, help would be coming back to them quickly. This is a very hard ask, but we saw very little organizational hoarding or hiding of materials or personnel. I firmly believe that is a testament to the trust developed between Renee and the VISN directors. We were able to continually demonstrate and sustain a model of operational agility unmatched in a continent-wide response.

Responding to a crisis that may occur once in a hundred years drew me to a book written in 2007 by Nassim Taleb entitled *The Black Swan*. Taleb describes "A Black Swan" event as an "unexpected event of large magnitude and consequence and their dominant role in history." [29] I had used this book in a number of speeches promoting the need for diversity in leadership teams experience. It was my belief that leadership teams need leaders drawn from different experiential backgrounds in order to ensure that there exists the ability within the team to respond to unexpected and unique events and challenges. A Black Swan, by definition, is something a leader has never seen before. Prior to COVID-19, all our systems were developed, staffed, and deployed with a regional challenge at the heart of the scenario. No one had ever considered a universal, continent-wide simultaneous challenge.

Another way to consider this Black Swan-type event is: What if every bit of your experience is not good enough to prepare you for what is about to happen to you or your organization? In preparation for the response to such an event, a leader should be surrounded by a leadership team that has a diverse set of skills and experience. Strong leadership teams require diversity of career experiences and backgrounds. The reader already knows that I am comfortable with combat-experienced Veterans. But we needed much more than that to respond to a once-in-a-hundred-year event. Luckily, we had recruited and developed a cohesive independent and collegial team that would face the next eighteen months of challenges. I am convinced that an event like this pandemic was a once-in-five-generations of leadership event, and therefore none of us was really prepared for the outcome or the challenge. Only a leadership team with broad diversity of skills and experiences could be successful. Even then, creating the correct leadership culture was essential.

The media is filled with Monday morning quarterbacks that will tell you they saw it coming and we should have been prepared more thoroughly. Those are the same "experts" that would tell you we wasted assets during the 2005 to 2016 eleven-year hurricane-free period in the continental United States when we maintained and grew emergency medical readiness for the inevitable next hurricane to hit the United States.

Diversity can be a fraught and controversial word today. There is, I believe, appropriately significant and nearly continuous discussion occurring about the ability of our nation to undo historical wrongs, done over the history of America to communities of color and to potentially give preference to various individuals based on those historical disadvantages. What I am discussing here in this instance, however, is something different but not mutually exclusive. I am referring to diversity of thought and diversity of experience. When building a team, I am always looking for individuals with different experience sets than my own.

This ensures to the greatest extent possible diversity of ideas during problem-solving. A leadership team that can respond to a Black Swan event must be diverse in thought. I worried during the initial phases of the pandemic when the leadership team began a senior leader decision brief regarding an impending challenge with the caveat "we all agree." My view immediately was that the right people are not at the table if there isn't at least one contrarian present. A contrarian is not an obstructionist. A contrarian is one who rejects the popular answer and provides another solution because they see something differently in the challenge before us.

That response is far different than an obstructionist who tells you all the reasons you're wrong in your approach and creates deliberate delay to process change or decision-making. An obstructionist is easily exposed by requesting that the obstructionist provide an alternative course of action. Usually, the answer is "just leave everything the same." The pandemic could have driven the VHA into a position of "sitting it out." The safe position would have been to argue that the risk to America's Veterans was too great, and we should preserve all of our capability for the Veteran. I felt that the aggressive spread of the disease did not provide us that luxury. In addition, the enormous skills of the VHA to care for critically ill patients were so unique that they must be brought to the benefit of all Americans.

As an aside, the nation's health delivery structure had few systems in place to regionally manage bed capacity and patient flow at this time. Because of this, there was minimal ability to effectively coordinate care between independent, often competing commercial delivery systems. Across most communities and regions, there was no unifying healthcare delivery governance or coordinating asset as could be provided by a system like the VHA. The ability of VHA to "see" the nation and its regions daily quickly revealed the profound weaknesses of healthcare delivery systems as they exist today. This weakness is not a criticism of their excellence in individual care delivery; it is directed to their inability to cooperatively share assets and integrate capability (during a national emergency) across silos cemented by competitive interaction between individual health systems.

Returning to the point of this chapter, leaders must draw contrarian thinkers out in any discussion. Renee Oshinski, as the leader of operations, was my best contrarian thinker. She would open each of those statements with, "I know you probably don't want to hear this, but . . ." She would then proceed to explain the risk of a course of action and always, once the dust cleared, she provided well thought-out solutions to reach the goal we were attempting to reach while reducing risk. In retro-spect, these were some of the most important challenges that I and the leadership team could hear. They either forced me and the team to defend the considered decision or, more commonly, make our amended decisions stronger with a greater likelihood of regional leader followership and, therefore, success. When I became concerned that I wasn't hearing every potential risk or second-order effect of a decision, or when there was just too much consensus, I finished each of those meetings with the following question, "Is there a contrarian in the room, or does anyone want to take a contrarian view?" A long pause, some-times uncomfortably so, would often occur, but it more often than not drew out those with something to add or improve our decisions.

There was another value in this approach to ensuring every voice is heard, and that is to create a sense of ownership by as many organizational leaders as possible in the ultimate deci-sion or the chosen course of action, even by those who had not spoken. There was a deliberate attempt at consensus building and, therefore, a greater likelihood of creating followership and adoption of the chosen course of action, and thus rapid move-ment toward success.

There is an additional final nuance to this discussion. How a senior leader responds to the contrarian has a lasting and profound effect on the entire team. I was working as a one-star Army general officer in a planning session with a very senior uniformed leader of the Army. We sequestered senior leaders for a day in a remote location to discuss some structural changes to Army maneuver units. Medical units were included for some reason that I still don't understand, but it was an extraordinary lesson in a lost leadership opportunity. The senior leader who was also facilitating the session began talking at the beginning of the four-hour session, and two and a half hours later, was still talking. In the last ninety minutes, he solicited input to what was clearly a completed decision. Every input or potential suggested refinement was met with dismissive responses by the senior leader until the room became quiet. This ended the session early, and the leader said in closing, "All of you now understand where we are going, and I expect you to be on board."

This senior leader had a chance to refine and improve a decision. He further had the chance to create adherence from those in attendance for the chosen approach and assess the intellectual capital of his leadership team as assembled. He denied himself all of those by his demeanor and approach. All of us have been in the room with leaders like this. The response is to put your head down and remain unnoticed. I believe that sessions like this are still extraordinarily common and reflect leaders that will never be able to respond to a Black Swan event. Inside the military, despite a flawed leader, uniformed service members of all branches will do everything possible to successfully complete a mission. Those tasks would be much easier to fulfill with leaders who honestly listened and acknowledged their subordinates' input in a respectful manner.

CHAPTER ELEVEN

Leveraging the Strategic National Stockpile, and Never Have One of Anything

THE LEADERSHIP OF THE federal health response to the rapidly evolving COVID-19 pandemic was coordinated by the Department of Health and Human Services (HHS). Within HHS is the Office of the Assistant Secretary for Preparedness and Response (ASPR). The mission of this office is stated in the HHS website as follows. The "ASPR leads the Nation's medical and public health preparedness for, response to, and recovery from disasters and public health emergencies." [30] The assistant secretary at the beginning of the pandemic was Dr. Robert Kadlec. Dr. Kadlec is a physician and Air Force Veteran and served as the ASPR from January 2017 until January 2021. He was experienced, thoughtful, and collaborative with a remarkable work history in biodefense. His service during this period was unfortunately marked by controversy after his demotion of an NIH scientist who led the Biomedical Advanced Research and Development Authority. I had dealt with Dr. Kadlec for years, and in multiple different venues and in all of my dealings with him and his team, he was a good and honest partner who, in the case of the pandemic, recognized the VHA for its pivotal role in the federal medical response.

Of note, the ASPR also controlled the nation's Strategic National Stockpile.

In 1998, Congress passed the Consolidated Appropriations Act that designated fifty-one million dollars to support the stockpiling of vaccines and pharmaceuticals at the CDC. This occurred after the publication of a fictional novel by Richard Preston entitled *The Cobra Event*. President Bill Clinton read the book in 1998, which details the actions of a fictional scientist who intentionally spread a virus throughout New York City. President Clinton was so moved by this fictional account that he convened a senior panel of scientists and cabinet officials to discuss the potential response and the nation's preparedness for such a scenario. By October 1998, the administration had requested, and Congress had passed, the enabling legislation and funding to support pharmaceutical and vaccine stockpiling under the leadership of the CDC. The legislation enabled the National Pharmaceutical Stockpile that evolved and was later renamed the Strategic National Stockpile (SNS) over ensuing administrations. Subsequent administrations expanded the stockpile to include protective personal equipment. As part of this evolution, control of the stockpile moved to the ASPR during the Trump administration. [31]

The Strategic National Stockpile exists to supplement state and local medical supplies during public health emergencies. In 2003, this pharmaceutical stockpile was supplemented by adding personal protective equipment and became jointly managed by Homeland Security and HHS. In 2001, the SNS was actually utilized in response to the attack on the World Trade Center on Sept 11th, and one week later that same year in the response to the anthrax attacks that continued until October 9th. During that nearly one-month period, five Americans died, and seventeen were sickened from exposure to anthrax that had arrived in mail delivered by the US Postal Service. The targets of these attacks were US Senators and media leaders. Since that time, the SNS has been used for regional responses to public health events, including Hurricane Katrina and Superstorm Sandy. In 2018, the Trump administration directed that the control of the SNS be moved under the ASPR. The SNS should be considered as a massive capability and its sustainment an impressive and complex task. Rapid depletion of this civilian-directed stockpile early in the pandemic and its ability to be resupplied created a demand on industry that would substantially affect the ability of VHA to sustain operations and fulfill its rapidly evolving mission. More on that later.

It is notable that the Federal Emergency Management Agency (FEMA) falls under the direction of the Department of Homeland Security and is responsible for on-the-ground support of disaster recovery. FEMA executes this mission by providing subject matter experts in specialized fields and funding of disaster recovery efforts, but FEMA is not composed of pandemic response health care experts as they are more focused on large scale but regional disasters, such as hurricanes, tornados, earthquakes, wildfires, and so on.

As the federal government began its response to the pandemic, the federal response was facing requests for emergent support from more than 114 state and tribal federal disaster declarations. In response to the rapid depletion of medical materials in these 114 areas, the president declared a public health emergency on March 13th of 2020. This declaration gave authority under what is called the Stafford Act for federal agencies to respond and support local agencies. The ASPR and VHA had already completed a number of VHA readiness discussions, and the ASPR understood well VHA's concerns and our unique capabilities.

Unfortunately, the federal response was complicated in its early days by interagency fragmentation between HHS and its subordinate CDC. It was further complicated by significant stress between DHS and its subordinate FEMA. The president, therefore, tasked Vice President Pence to ensure the alignment of these federal agencies in their response. The vice president convened a committee of federal agencies to respond to this task. Tragically, the nation's largest federal health care system, VHA, was not included in the vice president's ad hoc committee. The secretary of the VA would not become a member of this group until much later and only after a conversation between VA Secretary Wilkie and the VP where the VA secretary articulated the challenges health delivery systems were experiencing.

Therefore, medical input to the vice president from this group would come primarily from public health specialists from the CDC, but not from those actually operating health-care delivery systems. My point in this is that both voices are absolutely needed for an effective response, and this is one of the key lessons learned in this phase of the pandemic. The voice of America's federal and civilian health care delivery systems have struggled to have their concerns for the sustainment of care delivery capability heard by our most senior leaders. This resulted in further fragmentation that the ASPR attempted to overcome by hosting regular coordination discussions between DOD, VHA, Indian Health, and the United States Public Health Service. VHA leaders found most of these efforts laudable but incredibly fragmented, and we quickly identified that developing a common operating picture was essential to our hoped-for coordinated federal response. The presence of a common operating picture (as provided by the VA health operations center) would identify the same challenges and predict the future that I have previously described. The presence of common challenges and gaps in capability would have driven all of us to a unified response.

It is welcome news that significant discussions are now occurring amongst congressional staff to strengthen the roll of the ASPR as the lead coordinator of federal health response. I believe that Congress should review these events and consider the implications of the 2012 Biodefense Act and Executive Order 13603 that controls the authorities of federal agency response to ensure all stakeholders are effectively heard in future pandemics for the benefit of the American people.

The fact that FEMA had never responded to this type of continent-wide public health emergency and was never envisioned or structured as a medical response agency complicated and slowed the response, in large part, due to naivete outside of the agency of what FEMA actually did. Despite these unanticipated weaknesses, FEMA should be recognized for rapid implementation of what would be called Project Airbridge, which delivered massive amounts of medical supplies, primarily from Pacific Rim (Asian) nations. These nations produce the majority of these supplies for the world. FEMA also effectively distributed those supplies across the nation, thus sustaining and basically rescuing the civilian healthcare delivery systems across the United States.

During the early stages of the pandemic, there remained significant debate about the safety of air travel. As the government debated telework and business travel, I continued traveling (on commercial aircraft) in order to ensure that we fully understood the challenges faced by our frontline employees.

This created an elaborate pre- and post-travel personal ritual as we worked to ensure we did not expose anyone to the virus at the travel destination and as I returned home. We developed, as a family, processes to protect members of my family. We were tested at every site we visited. Not only did this give us a modicum of safety, but it also gave me an opportunity to lead by example and meet the extraordinary staff who were manning the testing clinics. We also tried to limit travel to those sites that would need minimal overnight stays as restaurants and food were often not available. When I returned home, we established a changing station in the garage at my home in order to change clothes and wipe down shoes, attempting to reduce the risk that I would carry the virus into our home. My wife laid out a plastic garbage bag that clothes were secured within. Shoes were sprayed and wiped with disinfectant, and I wiped all exposed skin surfaces with hand sanitizer before I proceeded directly to a shower. This was an important reminder of the fear and precautions every employee of every medical center was experiencing every single day.

Once we established all of these protocols, primarily obtained from frontline workers on how they were protecting their own families, I traveled in early June 2020 to the city of Chicago. I completed this trip to the Hines VAMC, where we had deployed a mobile intensive care unit. This was new technology manufactured for VHA by a company in Florida. We had deployed it to Chicago as a proof-of-concept event. The capabilities of the ICU included the unique ability for the twenty-bed facility to generate and purify its own water and concentrate its own oxygen. This type of sophisticated technology was going to be necessary in order to meet the demand for critical care beds across the nation. Our plan was to field at least one of these units in each of four geographic quadrants of the continental United States. This would facilitate rapid deployment. The technology was so unique that there was significant media attention at the event, and we were able to meet with regional FEMA leadership who were particularly interested in the technology and the capabilities of VHA. I found these regional FEMA leaders highly experienced and thoughtful, and they expressed a willingness to partner with regional VHA assets in potential future needs. In response to this meeting, during our next daily operations center update, we encouraged local VISN leaders to contact regional FEMA leaders in order to overcome what I found was significant fragmentation of the interagency response in Washington, DC, where there remained little knowledge and understanding of each other's capabilities even months into the pandemic response.

Daily coordination meetings with the ASPR, HHS, DOD, and FEMA occurred at the FEMA command center in Washington, DC. Our representative was Dr. Steve Lieberman, then serving as the principal deputy under secretary for health, the number-two executive for VHA reporting directly to the office of the under secretary for health (executive in charge). Steve and I agreed that he was the most knowledgeable of the capabilities of the VHA and that he should attend these interagency coordination meetings in person and on a daily basis. His express direction was to provide an empowered VHA decision maker to the "mission" assignment discussion that occurred at FEMA and ensure that a VHA official who thoroughly understood VHA capabilities was present for all discussions. "Missions" were formal requests for help from governors or tribal leaders to support their local facilities with personnel or equipment, and VHA was able to offer support where we could. Steve was empowered to commit the VHA system and its regions to missions that he believed we could execute with a significant probability of success and limited disruptions to Veteran care.

Steve Lieberman is trained and board certified as a critical care physician who has accumulated an extraordinary understanding of critical care medicine but also of federal disaster response and public health emergencies over his more than thirty years of federal service at the VHA. He has deployed as a provider for VHA in previous regional public health emergencies and was the obvious choice as my deputy for this work. In addition, his calm demeanor, ability to ask probing questions that reveals otherwise hidden risks, and a presentation style as a knowledgeable professional can command a room of strong personalities. Steve's efforts to ensure the interagency community fully understood what VHA could and could not accomplish and articulate our commitment to grow capability throughout the pandemic were essential to the interagency recognition of our potential role and to facilitate our successful response to all assigned missions. In a zero-defect mission, we could not have asked for a better advocate.

Coincident to these centralized daily meetings in Washington, DC, we began to hear from local health system leaders that the commercial health systems that surrounded VHA facilities needed help. These calls were generated by civilian health system leaders directly to our nearby medical centers' leadership teams. The calls were desperate, especially in NYC, where hospitals were overwhelmed with critically ill and dying patients. Unfortunately, it was not as easy as just saying, "send us your patients," as the ability to spend congressionally appropriated dollars specifically appropriated for Veterans on civilians literally required a specific and detailed request from a state-elected governor to the president of the United States. The president would then need to accept the request (a process completed by FEMA and HHS) and, only then, under the authority of the Stafford Act, VHA or another federal agency could respond. The process of making this happen quickly became a full-time engagement for Steve as he mentored local leaders on how to contact their governor's public health experts and submit their requirements. This was often complicated by state government policy makers and governor's advisors inexperienced in generating requests for federal aid that would successfully pass their governor's most senior team of advisors. Once the request came to the president, the federal government had to develop systems that quickly propagated a mission assignment potentially to the VHA. Once this system was completed, federal funds could be used to support those in need.

I found this entire system unreasonably slow and complex, and it violated my basic concept to allow the frontline leaders to manage this process. Unfortunately, violation of the Stafford Act processes carries significant financial and legal penalties, and throughout this unwieldy process, patients were accumulating in hallways and emergency rooms across the affected community. Calls between clinical leadership of VHA and surrounding hospitals became increasingly desperate, especially in NYC, and we did what we could to help them navigate the process as quickly as possible.

Steve, a relentless optimist, and tireless worker, was essential in this response, and we decided that once there was at least a 60-percent chance of mission assignment that we would begin moving VHA assets and accepting critically ill non-Veteran patients into our facilities. This process was amazingly frustrating to all involved, and all of us believed it left patients at risk. But nevertheless, we had to try.

Dr. Joan McInerney, the New York regional VISN leader, was able to overcome the administrative barriers primarily because of the long-term relationships she and her medical center directors had with local health system leaders across this region. In addition, the sheer experience of these leaders and the VHA's well-known ability to care for critically ill patients enabled us to accept the first non-Veteran critically ill patients to the New York and New Jersey VHA hospitals by late March 2020. This monumental accomplishment was possible only because of the extraordinary diligence of these leaders. It was further facilitated by the fact that there were established relationships at multiple professional levels between providers in VHA and the civilian health care community.

Future nationwide pandemic or widespread health emergency response must recognize the need to develop improved and simplified processes and relationships between delivery systems that ensure the orderly transfer of critically ill patients. The easy approach to this type of work would unload the minimally sick patients from an institution and avoid transfer of the critically ill. In the case of this pandemic, that approach was not possible because of the sheer volume of critically ill patients and the huge demand these very complex patients placed on the hospital infrastructure.

An example of this was the reports beginning to emerge from Europe, where hospital oxygen delivery systems were failing because of high oxygen flow rates, thus resulting in massive ice formation occurring on the exposed oxygen piping and slowing oxygen flow to patients. VHA engineers began to work possible solutions to this potential catastrophic failure and develop alternative oxygen delivery systems should primary delivery systems fail. This falls under the category of "never have one of anything" in a crisis, and obviously infrastructure like this is not easy to duplicate. Soon, virtually every VHA medical center had large oxygen cylinders in the corners of each COVID-19 patient care room to protect patients from potential catastrophic failure of the centralized system.

CHAPTER TWELVE

The Secretary and Congressional Leadership

O VER MY MILITARY AND civilian government career, I have worked with many servant leaders who were political appointees from both political parties. I have found all but a small minority to be extraordinarily committed to the mission of their agencies, and they delivered accomplished skill to the performance of their assigned positions. As a former military officer, I consistently attempted to avoid partisanship in every possible decision. When asked privately about my political affiliation, I would often say the following, "I am aligned mostly with John Adams' comments about political parties. He wrote in a letter to his wife Abigail that the problem with political parties is, eventually, they place party interests before the needs of the Republic." I am sure I paraphrased my response and did not do justice to the words of one of the founding leaders of the nation. I have always believed that whatever partisanship I express should be directed to the benefit of the American Veteran and uniformed service members and their families. It is my hope that my actions and years of service reflected that consistent partisanship.

We were fortunate during the time of the pandemic to have the leadership of Secretary Robert Wilkie as the tenth secretary of Veterans Affairs. The secretary was extraordinarily experienced and well known to the White House, interagency space, and on Capitol Hill. He operated under some clear and direct leadership principles.

The soon-to-be-confirmed secretary introduced himself to me when I had asked for a discussion with him just before his confirmation and before I accepted government reemployment in the role of leading VHA. I was not yet an employee of VHA and wanted to ensure that my vision for the future of VHA aligned with the soon-to-be-confirmed secretary's vision. In addition, I wanted to ensure that we would be able to work together for the benefit of Veterans. We met in the Pentagon, where the secretary continued to serve in his Senate-confirmed position as DOD under secretary for Personnel and Readiness until his Senate confirmation to become secretary of the VA came to pass.

The secretary nominee began the conversation by pointing out that his conversation with me as a private citizen in no way presumed his confirmation by the Senate. He then paused to listen. He was gracious with his time and attention in listening to my vision to transform VHA based on three pillars of transformation. First, restore the trust of the American Veteran and the American people and their elected representatives in the VHA. This would be achieved by transforming VHA into what is referred to as a high reliability organization. Second, for the VHA to become a learning organization. This pillar has been reviewed at length in previous chapters. Third, to modernize all of our operating systems upon which we managed the VHA. The centerpiece of modernization would be the electronic medical record tracking system transition from a homegrown VHA system called VISTA to a commercial off-the-shelf system.

The fielding of a new electronic health record (EHR) in a health system forces that health system to reexamine virtually all its business processes. The EHR should be viewed as a platform upon which all other operating systems connect in order to run the health care system. For example, the supply chain operating system and financial operating systems would also need to be modernized as we moved to this new clinical tool. The coordination of these modernization efforts would be a monumental undertaking across what I believed would be a decade of work.

Upon completing what was about a forty-five-minute brief, the secretary nominee shook my hand. He said he was anxious to work with me, and then he said the following, "I am not of your world, Dr. Stone. I am not a doctor. If confirmed, I will need you to tell me how I need to support this vision of the future, and I will do all I can do to bring this to fruition."

The secretary (following confirmation) always deferred to subject matter expertise. This is not to infer that he lacked his own vision. He wanted Veterans to trust the VA. He wanted Veterans to choose the VA for their benefits and care. He believed in the unique role of VHA in American health care and its key role in the education of future American health care providers. He visibly supported VA research and elevated our successful partnership with industry and academic partners in ways that would become evident early in the pandemic. He was most extraordinary in his willingness to roll up his sleeves and work to ensure the VA's success.

As the pandemic ravaged the population of the southern portions of New York State in March and April 2020, we sought counsel and guidance from Secretary Wilkie, who had since been confirmed for his position as secretary in July 2018. We discussed the interagency challenges that we were facing. We described for him the difficulty in operating within the convoluted interagency environment while pressed for timely and agile support from local medical leaders with seriously ill patients desperate for care. We also discussed the challenge that no health delivery system had a voice at the vice president's COVID-19 task force. The secretary acknowledged our concerns and immediately engaged in correcting those challenges we had described for him. Within twenty-four hours, he sought and garnered support from the vice president to join the president's COVID-19 task force chaired by Vice President Pence on a permanent basis.

The secretary also came to us with a proposal that he would call every governor in the country to pledge VA's and his personal support for their states. In this manner, he would prepare and partner with governors to respond rapidly to the requests for support from their individual state's health care leadership. He would further ensure that each governor would have access to the secretary himself and thus would facilitate the rapid provision of care for each state's citizens. He promised each of them that any problems or challenges that might arise, he would be directly available to each of those governors. At the conclusion of our meeting, the secretary suspended his other work and began calling every governor. Every one of them answered or returned his calls except two, one who happened to be from my home state of Michigan and the second, the governor of New York. Regardless of party affiliation, all forty-eight to whom he spoke were gracious and appreciative of his and the VA's effort to support them. They also universally acknowledged the

Secretary's personal pledge of support to their efforts to help in the protection of their state's population. Over the next year, the VHA would support hundreds of mission requests from forty-eight states to include the states of Michigan and New York. The Michigan mission was in support of the Detroit area and included provision of critical care beds within the Detroit and Ann Arbor VAMCs. We also supplied a mobile pharmacy to the Detroit convention center at COBO hall, which was being converted to a pop-up hospital. As part of deploying that asset, a telephonic conversation between the secretary and the governor of Michigan eventually occurred to discuss deployment timelines. The Michigan support was substantially enabled by the diligent effort and the long-standing relationships between those Michigan-based VHA medical center directors and the VISN director, Rima Nelson, whose willingness to make decisions and move forward was a model for all leaders.

I firmly believe the secretary's sustained and personal engagement effort was instrumental in saving countless lives and opened a previously nonexistent channel of communication with the myriad of states requesting VHA support. His commitment also demonstrated to VHA field leaders his alignment and support of their heroic efforts. He began attending our daily operations center updates at this time in order to listen and express support and build what I believe were lasting and impactful relationships with the VISN and medical center directors in the midst of this crisis. His willingness to roll up his sleeves and work to ensure our success was extraordinary.

He would speak during HOC national briefings about what he had heard from the governors to include their concerns, thus allowing regional VISN leaders to adjust their readiness posture to respond more quickly. The secretary actively engaged

both through phone calls and personal visits with other cabinet secretaries to resolve problems between agencies. He made
personal visits to FEMA and HHS to break down barriers in
communication and emphasize his willingness to resolve any
issue that would prevent VA from emerging as a full and productive partner to HHS and FEMA. The secretary fully supported the proposed assignment of multiple senior executives
from VHA to FEMA to include medical supply chain experts
to help resolve rapidly emerging challenges. These individuals
were welcomed by FEMA and HHS because the secretaries of
HHS, Homeland Security, and the VA were visibly engaged and
aligned in their federal response.

I remained concerned with interagency health care capabilities and the ability to sustain the response capacity of the
federal health provider network. For example, DOD operates
a medical care delivery system that has been severely strained
by the Global War on Terrorism and had repeatedly deployed
and engaged most of the uniformed medical force structure
since September 11, 2001. I personally knew most of the DOD
medical leaders well and was aware of their unwavering commitment to the American people and the mission to support
those Americans in need. The DOD was, during this time, however, being repeatedly called upon by senior political leaders
for extraordinary amounts of providers in an effort to rapidly field missions like the Navy hospital ships Comfort and
Mercy moving to each coast. In addition, they were deploying
smaller individual teams to support the temporary hospitals
being erected in cities around the nation. Should these demands
be sustained, the ability to remain wartime ready as a military
medical system would be challenged. I absolutely believed
DOD was on the verge of being unable to sustain their current

health care mission to provide routine care to US uniformed service members and their families if they were tasked further during the initial few months of the pandemic. I was also eager to have VHA assets employed as an effective partner to each of these agencies.

The nation's leaders need to reconsider the role of the federal health delivery system (to include DOD) in this type of domestic health care response mission that require large numbers of professional providers. Clear lines of responsibility between DOD, Public Health Service (PHS), Indian Health Service (IHS), and VHA need to be established. Very few actually are aware that the VHA's health care delivery system is about three times greater in size than DOD's. Guidelines, contingency planning, and sustained contingency plans need to be established and rehearsed in order to ensure future balanced use of these assets. The presence of these plans would ensure there is no degradation of any agencies' primary mission capability during a crisis. As part of this development, there should be a balance between agencies with increased clarity of VHA's responsibilities and capacity for a fourth mission response. The ASPR is the obvious integrating office in HHS to foster this potential partnership between the agencies that would clearly define all agencies' responsibility in future public health emergencies.

As the breadth and depth of the spread of the pandemic began to advance across the nation, I was asked in early March 2020 to provide testimony to the House Veterans Affairs Committee, chaired by Congressman Mark Takano (Democrat). The chairman has been representing California's 41st district since 2013. Following the conclusion of the testimony, the chairman asked to speak with me privately. He began the conversation with: "Dr. Stone, what will the VHA need for resources to respond to the pandemic on behalf of the American people and the American Veteran population?" I was dumbfounded. The VHA's budget already contained substantial funds for emergency response operations that I have previously described.

The amount of congressionally appropriated dollars a department receives is the result of complex negotiations between cabinet secretaries and the president's budget leaders. These requests are then submitted to Congress as part of the president's annual official budget request. Congress then passes a budget, and funds flow to the department. In no way could a leader at my level bypass the VA secretary and the president of the United States and ask for emergency funds without their knowledge and support. I looked at the chairman after an uncomfortable pause on my part and said , "Mr. Chairman, you and your committee on both sides of the aisle have provided the VHA with adequate resources in the yearly appropriation to cover our needs. We are prepared for what will come, and we will ensure all Veterans and the American people are cared for."

What came next stunned me despite my many years of dealing with Congress and congressional leaders. The chairman said the following, "Dr. Stone, I absolutely believe that you are underestimating the severity of the crisis that is about to overtake you. I want you to think long and hard about your response and call me tomorrow with an early estimate of your needs. This Congress is going to ensure you have the resources for whatever might happen in advance." I thanked the chairman and returned to VA central office. In my now nearly thirty-five years of government service, I have never encountered an elected official who so sincerely saw the "Black Swan" that was coming and understood its potential implications.

Upon my return to VA Central Office, I went to see Secretary Wilkie, who had an open-door policy for any leader's concerns or challenges. I related the conversation between Chairman Takano and myself. We discussed the chairman's request and agreed to develop some worst-case scenarios. As we put together potential scenarios, we could immediately see a possible need for 17 million dollars in additional emergency operational funds. This type of out-of-cycle budget requests are sent from VHA to the secretary, who shares it with the White House. The White House then adjusts as necessary and considers the implications of these requests and forwards them to Congress. The VA request morphed into 70 million dollars by the time it reached Congress, as it included funds for not just VHA but the entire VA. This also reflects the rapidly evolving spread of the virus and the rapid escalation of material cost as worldwide demand for medical material skyrocketed. When the pandemic response comprehensive CARES Act legislation was passed by Congress, that would provide financial relief to broad sectors of the American economy, VHA was budgeted within the legislation to receive an additional 15.8 billion dollars (with a B!).

The ultimate number (of 15.8 billion) came because of the rapidly evolving vision and significant government experience of four House and Senate leaders. In the House of Representatives, Chairman Mark Takano (Democrat) and Ranking Member Phil Roe (Republican, now retired) represented the House Veterans Affairs oversight committee leadership. Chairman Takano is Harvard educated and had spent twenty years as a public-school teacher before running for and being elected to Congress. Congressman Roe had served in Congress since 2009, representing Tennessee's 1st Congressional District. He had been chairman of the House Veterans Affairs Committee from 2017 to 2019. He is an Army Veteran and a retired obstetrics and gynecology physician.

On the Senate side, the Senate Veterans Affairs Committee was chaired by Jerry Moran (Republican), the senior senator from the state of Kansas. He has held office since 2011 and had previously served Kansas' 1st Congressional District for fourteen years in the House. The ranking member (Democrat) of the Senate Veterans Affairs Committee at that time was Jon Tester. The reader has already been introduced to Senator Tester in my discussion of the MISSION Act implementation. He was elected to the Senate in 2007 and continues with his family to operate his family farm in the state of Montana.

The American Veteran owes a great debt to the vision and passion of these four long-serving elected leaders and their deeply experienced staff, who provided extraordinary and historic emergency funding to VHA. Each of them ensured their individual caucuses were informed and that the funding was rapidly available. The early availability of this significant funding allowed VHA to purchase more than 6000 additional ventilators, four mobile intensive care units, and multiple wheeled care and command center vehicles that guaranteed a robust COVID-19 VHA emergency response. In addition, and of extraordinary importance, we were able to financially incentivize the rapid hiring of more than 80,000 VHA employees over the remainder of the 2020 calendar year as the pandemic accelerated across the nation. These newly hired employees replaced those who retired or left, in part due to the personal risk of bedside delivery of COVID-19 health care. In addition, we were able to stabilize and rapidly grow the workforce to accommodate the growth of 4000 acute care VHA beds. This ability to stabilize the workforce was key to our ability to rapidly take on missions across the nation where civilian care was at risk of being overwhelmed. All of this was only possible because these four congressional leaders took financial constraints off the table for VHA and allowed us to fully exercise our Veteran care and fourth mission capability. My distaste for politics will always be softened by this experience in which true problem-solving and collaboration occurred quickly in order to serve the needs of the nation. I would add that the congressional staff of this leadership team are extraordinary Americans and, more truly, unsung heroes in this fight.

What I have just described reflects an example of congressional oversight committees working in a bipartisan basis for a single goal, the well-being of America's Veterans and the American people. From my viewpoint, this is how Congress should work and provides a glimpse of what could be accomplished if all of Congress worked together like these four leaders, committee members, and their staff.

This congressional leadership also enabled the ability of Secretary Wilkie to determine the actual number of acute care beds that VHA would ultimately dedicate to the emerging national civilian health care crisis. The VHA's first and nonnegotiable mission is always to provide care for America's Veterans. We knew that we must preserve adequate beds for every Veteran who might present to us for care. We also knew that with the shortage of civilian hospital beds in many communities that Veterans who had never enrolled in VHA health care would likely come to us for care.

It is notable that of America's nearly twenty million Veterans, only about 9.5 million have enrolled in VHA health care. About 85 percent of America's Veterans have health insurance through their post-government service civilian employer. Even most of those who come to VHA for care have other health insurance. Many of those who do not enroll believe that they are not sick or disabled enough to deserve care provided by VHA. The most frequent answer from an unenrolled Veteran to the question of "Why did you never enroll in VHA health care?" is the following: "There are service members who were hurt way worse than me. I don't want to take their spot." Many Veterans' families finally seek care for their Veteran for end-of-life issues or problems with cognitive decline when a family can no longer care for their Veteran. The Veteran-specific integrated care available to Veterans through the VHA provides significant value to identifying and caring for service-related problems from Agent Orange, mental health, military sexual trauma, airborne hazard exposure, and so on. Our concern was that large numbers of unenrolled Veterans would enroll during the COVID-19 pandemic due to the lack of civilian hospital beds or available civilian-provided care. Any additional enrollment could challenge the availability of our growing capacity to provide care.

In order to predict future care demand, we began tracking the prevalence of COVID-19 across Veteran populations and discovered that Veterans enrolled in VHA health care, although significantly older than the non-Veteran American population, were experiencing COVID-19 infection rates that was lower than the rest of American citizens. In addition, the percentage of COVID-19-positive Veteran patients hospitalized and dying was also lower than the civilian population. The average age of an American is thirty-eight years old. The average age of an American veteran is fifty-eight years old. As we learned more about what was occurring around the world in our daily reports, the patient's age and the presence of comorbid medical conditions created risk for hospitalization and higher rates of death from COVID-19. Obviously, we couldn't change age. We, therefore, hypothesized that the comprehensive medical management of hypertension, diabetes, and all other comorbid conditions for patients cared for in the VHA system was at a significantly more effective level of disease control than patients cared for in the rest of the US health care system. This enhanced control of these medical conditions reduced the risk of hospitalization and death from COVID-19 in Veterans when matched against an age-matched cohort of American non-Veterans.

There was thus an inherent advantage of enrolling in a fully integrated health care system such as the VHA. There are few health systems in the United States that are fully integrated and incentivize lifetime health promotion and disease control in an effort to prevent hospitalization and the complications of chronic disease. VHA's assessment of quality indicators for evidence of the control of these diseases in enrolled patients are significantly higher when compared to most of the nation's community care delivery systems. These can be found in tracking programs like the CMS (Medicare)-sponsored "Hospital Compare" rating system. Multiple independent studies have also confirmed the validity of the previous assertion. One example is the 2018 study of 121 health care markets that contained at least one VA medical center and a civilian hospital, conducted by Dartmouth Institute for Health Policy, and published in the Annals of Internal Medicine.[32] This study utilized Hospital Compare data and demonstrated that VA hospitals provided the "best" care in most of those 121 regions. Notable findings include "best" rankings in most markets for heart attack, heart failure, and pneumonia care.

CHAPTER THIRTEEN

Models of Care and Patient Transport

AS WE GREW THE VHA capacity for care and began to bring the 4000 additional beds to operational readiness, we actually began to experience decreases in enrolled Veteran hospitalization. This occurred as elective medical procedures were delayed and reduced in an effort to avoid COVID-19 spread and maintain available bed capacity. The secretary at that time made the decision to pledge 1500 of the newly operational beds to civilian (non-Veteran) capacity expansion. These beds would be made available preferentially to high intensity, complex, and, therefore, critically ill civilian patients. We would preserve a little over 60 percent of the newly created beds for possible surge demand from enrolled or newly enrolled Veterans.

In addition, we would vary by local community need the number of beds made available rather than designate a fixed number of beds for civilian use in each VHA hospital. This would provide maximum agility for patient flow and maximum community benefit in each VHA medical center. The secretary presented this increased critical care capacity model to HHS and FEMA, and there was immediate acceptance of his offer. Steve Lieberman was tasked to ensure that there was clear and transparent communication at all levels of government to include VHA leaders on potential civilian missions that could consume this available VHA critical care capacity.

Since the vice president-led COVID-19 task force was staffed with public health experts and not experts in health care delivery, the sheer magnitude of the secretary's announcement to the VP's task force and the effort it had taken to deliver this volume of critical care capacity was met with understandable indifference and a polite "thank you." The tasking for this newly available backstop for the American health care system would come through HHS and FEMA, so the actual response of the VP-led presidential COVID-19 task force had little effect on VHA operations.

A primary lesson learned for future government leaders is the recommendation to create a health delivery coordination council under the direction of the ASPR in HHS. The formation of this suggested council acknowledges the hugely disparate and uncoordinated care delivery models in the United States. Most civilian health systems operate completely independently of other providers in their communities and actively compete with geographically collocated hospital systems. The idea that all competition would somehow dissolve when the pandemic hit was operationally unreasonable and naïve. Even at the time of publishing of this book, the operational concerns of health care delivery systems are not well heard by senior federal government leaders, and this results in delays and even impedes potential support to the American people when a crisis strikes. The author acknowledges the development during the pandemic of a mission assignment council under the direction of the ASPR. The formal development, expansion, and sustainment of this capability would reduce future delays in support to Americans in need.

The VHA accepted a mission to support NYC hospitals on the 27th of March 2020 and accepted the first non-Veteran COVID-19 patient transfer into a VHA hospital in the city of New York. Critically ill and therefore complex patient transfers between institutions require significant communication and preplanning between providers and the transporting entity. While serving in Afghanistan, the model for the transport of critically ill and wounded from the battlefield included the delivery of a wounded service member to a trauma care unit (Forward Surgical Team or Combat Support Hospital) within one hour.

The concept of a post injury "golden hour" is a well-known trauma care principle that reflects primarily the challenge of sudden trauma-induced death from blood loss in those patients where blood replacement and the ability to stop additional hemorrhages are essential foundational principles. Simplified, the concept is delivering a patient to definitive care within an hour of injury. A wounded service member who arrives alive at a US military combat support hospital has more than a 96-percent chance of survival regardless of the severity of injury. The key to this very high survival rate is effective forward (battlefield) stabilization and then rapid movement to definitive care facilities, such as the US Army hospital in Landstuhl, Germany, as soon as possible.

This operating principle employed in the war in Afghanistan and Iraq was dramatically different than the WWII model of prolonged care and the establishment of actual rehabilitation hospitals in the European and Pacific theaters, where literally thousands of patients occupied hospital beds that were established in those combat theaters. Wounded service members were returned to frontline service after what could have been even a month or more of care and rehabilitation.

The newer model of care delivery employed in Afghanistan and Iraq since 2001 also reflected the historical lesson in previous wars that infectious disease would far outweigh actual combat wounds. The WWII model of combat health care delivery (large numbers of long-term beds near the battlefield) would be abandoned after Operation Desert Storm in the early 1990s. In planning and executing that short war, the US military deployed huge amounts of medical assets that went, thankfully, unused. The low usage also reflected the dramatic advances in air transport medicine provided in platforms like the C17, where the complex equipment of an actual intensive care unit could be installed within the plane's cargo space in a few hours. These advances resulted in the creation of a care delivery system in Afghanistan (and then later in Iraq) with an austere number of beds positioned far forward in the battlefield with the capability to stabilize and then rapidly transport casualties to Landstuhl, where an Army advanced trauma hospital has operated for many decades. Further transport of critically injured service members would then occur back to Walter Reed Military Medical Center or another military hospital most appropriate for the patient's needs.

At each of these transfers, an Air Force critical care air transport team would arrive and evaluate the patient for transfer and assess the stability of the patient to survive high altitude pressurization. That evaluation would include ensuring the appropriate supplies were available for a flight that would exceed ten hours. My point in reviewing all of this is that this type of professional interaction between providers does not normally exist in the civilian medical care system in the United States except for pediatric or neonatal intensive care transport and some rotary wing air ambulances usually owned by trauma centers.

This weakness in critical care patient transfer became apparent very early in the movement of patients from civilian to VHA hospitals across the country. Even with the availability of robust telemedicine or technology-enabled consultation between hospital critical care specialists and nurses, transfer of patients with complex ventilator needs was difficult. In response to this systemic weakness, most VHA medical centers designated a single critical care provider to assimilate all the information on a potential patient transfer in order to ensure all essential care information was captured and thus reduce the risk to the patient during and following transfer. In addition, the sophistication of the civilian medic and limitations in (state licensed) scope of practice rules in the handling of very ill ventilated patients during transport was dramatically different than the combat-hardened uniformed medic scope of practice of the US military. Because of that difference, it was not unusual for a critical care professional nurse from the transferring hospital to physically participate in vehicle-based care during transport and conduct face-to-face handoff to VHA providers immediately following the patient's arrival at the VHA. This consumption of critically short nursing assets was noted as an unanticipated strain on nursing staffing by receiving and transferring facilities. There are some robust learning messages in all of this. The American civilian ground ambulance systems need to ensure that civilian paramedics can work to the top of their licenses, and the restrictions on those licenses need to recognize the extraordinary success of the military model of medic-led care delivery by the heroic uniformed combat medic.

As the "golden hour" concept has developed and matured, the idea of rapid arrival of a patient transport vehicle and then rapid transport to a hospital (or from one hospital to another) has been called the "scoop and run" model of care. This model of scoop and run is not employed in many western European countries. This model is also very difficult to execute in rural areas of America, where rural hospitals rarely have the expertise and capable assets to intervene in the complex care of a critically ill or trauma victim. This has resulted in the recognition that patient survival after injury is often more about where you live (or were injured) than how quickly an ambulance transport can arrive. As rural hospitals across America continue to close or reduce services due to financial instability and thus reduce available capability in rural communities, the emergency medical response system of this nation needs to be reexamined.

There are other models of care transport.

On June 8, 2003, a suicide car bomber struck and destroyed a German military bus, killing four German soldiers and injuring twenty-nine in downtown Kabul, Afghanistan. The blast occurred at 8:30 am on a brilliantly clear morning. The bus was carrying German soldiers from their military base, where these soldiers had supported the International Security Assistance Force in support of Operation Enduring Freedom to Kabul International Airport for their return to Germany, having completed their mission. Kabul was, at that time, a chaotic city, and the streets were narrow and lined with multiple two- and three-story buildings. The roadways were filled with vehicles, and there were few operating traffic signals. It was not unusual during this time for low-flying coalition military aircraft to be targeted by small arms fire. In addition, traffic was often congested and even stopped. Vehicles were often unable to move, causing coalition forces to use vehicles equipped with heavy steel bumpers on the front and rear to push stopped vehicles out of the way and thus reduce the exposure of coalition soldiers to attack. The operating principle was that if your vehicle was stopped in traffic with vehicles in front and behind you, your chance of dying in an attack would increase exponentially. In response to this, the US military ran a scoop-and-run operation for US casualties throughout this area. Primarily executed by Black Hawk helicopters, the removal of a casualty was executed quickly and with the support of Apache heavily-armed attack helicopters, who provided defensive overwatch in case of attack during the retrieval of the injured. An Apache is a narrow fuselage helicopter that is heavily armed and able to deliver a precise response from low altitude to a myriad of threats.

Because of the large number of casualties in the German bus bombing (at least twenty-nine victims) and the extraordinary risk of an additional or secondary attack on the responding forces, the decision was made by the US air medical evacuation leadership to support casualty movement with a giant US Army CH-47 Chinook helicopter. These two rotor heavy-lift helicopters have been in service since 1961. They are big, but a single lift could move large numbers of patients very quickly. Army Chinook pilots can land the back of the helicopter on a building's flat roof and open the rear-loading ramp to onboard significant cargo and personnel rapidly and safely. The commitment of this asset was to attempt to reduce the number of repeat landings a Blackhawk crew would need to conduct and therefore clear the bombing site of injured quickly and thus reduce the crew's risk of attack.

When the first Chinook arrived at the bombing site with its Apache helicopter gunships in overwatch position, the Germans had already established a trauma-clearing location and even had erected a tent to keep the casualties out of the sun. The German commanding medical officer on the ground ordered our Chinook personnel to land and shut off the helicopter as they were going to stabilize the wounded prior to transport. For US personnel, this stabilization would be done during transport to a combat hospital. This "sit and wait" concept was completely foreign to the culture and training of the US evacuation team and considered by the personnel in the aircraft to be high risk to the responding American personnel and aircraft. The American leadership, therefore, extracted the helicopter and returned the aircraft and personnel to a safe nearby location until the Germans were ready to transport. The majority of the Germans injured were eventually transported by the international coalition-provided armored wheeled military ambulances, but a substantial number were eventually air transported.

The failure of the combined international medical team (to include the US) to recognize and understand the fundamental cultural differences that existed in trauma care response protocols of each coalition country resulted in substantial confusion and inefficiency that could have led to additional lives being lost. We resolved, in the hours following this devastating attack, to quickly review and reach concurrence on future mass casualty response within ISAF and the US-deployed health care teams. We rapidly reached an understanding on the commitment of combat military health care air and ground evacuation assets following this event. The German system had in fact delivered substantial value and, in all likelihood, reflected the movement of ER physicians and trauma surgeons to the patients at the bombing site, in spite of the risk to these rare and highly skilled personnel. The presence of a ambulance based physician or advanced practice nurse arriving at a trauma site or even a patient's home is not unusual in many European countries. This usually occurs by assigning a provider to an ambulance in those countries. The presence of these providers reduces the need for transport to hospitals and ensures appropriate triage of patients to the correct level of care. Significant care by these providers is delivered in the home, often obviating the need for transport altogether. This model of care has not been accepted in the United States.

We faced the same challenges as we attempted to move COVID-19 patients from civilian to VHA facilities, although not so dramatic. There are cultural and communication differences that must be overcome while developing trust and transparency between civilian, DOD, and other federal medical care delivery systems. Those skills must be practiced, and those professional relationships developed and sustained in advance of future public health challenges. We found that the VHA health system has significant capability in emergency operations at every medical center that is robust and routinely practiced, but the ability to communicate with civilian hospitals is completely relationship dependent and often was based on someone knowing the cell phone number of a civilian hospital leader. This weakness should be corrected in future crisis responses. I believe the development of an interfacility medical communication system in every American community is essential to this recommended transformation, not just for large pandemics but also for coordination of large-scale events, such as a bus accident or train derailment that can quickly overwhelm a single hospital or community.

The future evolution of ambulance transport in the US should acknowledge and consider the European model of including nurse (APRN) or physician providers on ambulances and thus reducing the frequency and risk of transport of a sick or injured patient. This model is most effective in response to illness that providers arriving to care for a patient can evaluate, diagnose, and complete the needed care at a patient's home and thus avoid the need for movement of the patient to a very costly emergency room unless absolutely necessary. The efficiency of this system should especially be considered in rural areas where hospital assets are austere and often at great distance from the patient's residence. (Success in this effort will depend upon the growth of what is defined as point-of-service testing of blood and body fluid specimens. And, in addition, that this technology is available in mobile settings.)

CHAPTER FOURTEEN

Looking For the Crystal Ball and Understanding the Aged Patient

THE AMERICAN HEALTH CARE system in the 1930s delivered physician provider-patient visits in the patient's home about 40 percent of the time. [33] Providers making house calls were routine and part of every physician's workday. As laboratory technology and imaging capability and technology advanced, patients were actually required to move from their homes to the lab and radiology services that had to be housed in facilities, usually within a hospital. The development of ever more complex technology within the brick-and-mortar footprint of community-based general hospitals has made access to care for marginalized populations a major challenge and has resulted in declining life spans and an enhanced disease burden for those communities (often communities of color) where the availability of care and the barrier of financial cost cannot be overcome. By the 1980s, less than 2 percent of physician-provided care was actually delivered by providers in patients' home. [34]

Much has been written by health-care delivery "experts" about the use of telemedicine platforms to connect providers and patients in an era where physically sending a provider to a patient's home seems unreasonable or inefficient (at least in the

United States). The major challenge remains the ability to deliver the laboratory and imaging technology (that forced this change in the last half of the twentieth century) to a patient's home and then the ability to connect those devices and the data from them in a readily accessible data retrieval platform. Much has also been written about providing common interchangeable electronic medical records. The key challenge, however, is to move these electronic record platforms beyond sophisticated word document retrieval and medical billing generation systems. Electronic medical record systems must transform into true patient-centered care delivery-enabling systems. The barrier to these advances and subsequent benefit to patients remains data capture from multiple disparate sources, such as diagnostic and imaging platforms and subsequent data management.

There are hundreds of commercial software programs attempting to capture a patient's data in the home, including everything from heart rhythm to temperature, and respiratory rate, oxygen saturation levels, and blood pressure are possible with minimal in-home equipment. Unfortunately, the transformative breakthrough to return substantial care to the home will not occur until we are remotely able to capture and analyze a blood or body fluid specimen with a high degree of accuracy. In addition, the development of delivered at-home, non-radiation-emitting imaging devices that are able to deliver diagnostic images remains elusive. Only when this level of technology is available will the probability of separating large numbers of patients from the current medical facility-based delivery model be significant.

The existing model of moving patients to a diagnostic facility has emerged over the last seventy years and consumed massive amounts of the nation's resources as well as patients' time. A willingness to embrace the change to non-facility based care will be further enabled by the availability of intelligent learning machines that can leverage and learn from worldwide repositories of patient data and outcomes. The connection of providers and patients, free of brick-and-mortar facilities, will be challenged (and even resisted) by a long-entrenched and highly profitable hospital business model that has been the centerpiece of massive health system investment and subsequent long-term health care system debt. This debt exists usually in the form of long-term investment bonds.

The American health care system and the VHA are at an inflection point in care. Increased amounts of care delivered in the home and away from institutions, enabled by substantial remote sensors and technology, will ultimately change what future leaders will encounter in the current facility-based American system. A patient-centric system of care delivery could substantially change the challenges health care leaders encounter in the next pandemic.

VHA has witnessed over many decades a progressive aging of Veteran patients. This patient aging has been associated with increased numbers of patients with cognitive decline in the Veteran population. This has occurred not only in Veterans but also across the entire American population. We should recognize that as much as 12 percent of all Americans suffer from some form of cognitive impairment as they age.[35] The presence of cognitive decline in a family member results in significant burden of care delivered by those patients' families. This burden of care falls especially on the Veterans' spouses, who most often serve as their in-home caregivers. In many severely compromised patients, the Veteran, unfortunately, either has no one willing to care for them, or their disease creates too heavy a physical or emotional burden on an aging spouse and family. The eventual movement of the Veteran to a long-term care facility typically becomes the next step in providing their ongoing health care.

The VHA operates a substantially different care model for these long-term care facilities and patients than the civilian medical system across the United States. The VHA long-term care facilities are often collocated with or even within VHA medical centers, allowing the movement of specialized personnel who are experts in geriatric care into and out of the facility each day. This occurs without disrupting the patients' safety or requiring vehicle movement of patients to an outside provider. In addition, common credentialling and privileging of providers in these facilities allows those who have cared for a Veteran for many years to continue their care, thus, avoiding the often-disruptive processes of turning a long-established patient's care over to a long-term care facility physician, who may be covering large numbers of patients. The VHA model is also strengthened by a heavy reliance on bedside professional nursing. In most civilian long-term care facilities, bedside care is provided by a nursing assistant with one professional nurse assigned to a care unit of twenty to forty patients. This model restricts the professional nurse's direct involvement in patient care. The professional nurse is limited to the creation or modification of patient care plans and the distribution of patient medications. There is little bedside care and interaction with patients by professional nurses in this model. The VHA long-term care delivery model, however, maintains a near acute care nursing to patient care staffing model with significant numbers of professional nurses at the bedside. This model is expensive, costing in excess of one hundred thousand dollars per patient per year for institutionalized long-term care. VHA can provide this model of care as a benefit without cost for Veterans who have sustained 70 percent or more in service-related disability or injury. This care model, however, is not within the financial reach of most non-service-disabled Veterans or non-Veteran Americans.

The VHA has also developed an in-home care delivery model for disabled Veterans that supports family caregivers and provides personnel and resources to enable Veterans to remain in their homes for as long as safely possible. A robust in-home system of support can cost about twenty-five thousand dollars per patient for effective care support each year. The ability of this in-home support delivered in order to delay or obviate the need to institutionalize a Veteran has significant financial cost avoidance to the VHA. In addition, there are few of us who, if given the choice, would fail to choose to stay in the familiar sur-roundings of our own homes and in the presence of our loved ones. As a result of these programs, more than two hundred thousand Veterans today are now cared for in their homes.

The profound relationship of America's Veterans to their individual states of residence goes back to the Revolutionary War when troops were generated on behalf of individual col-onies. That model continued into and through the Civil War when units were even designated as a numbered unit with the state's name. For example, Civil War service was provided by volunteers of the 16th Michigan Infantry Regiment. [36] This his-tory resulted in individual states funding and building congre-gate care Veteran homes in order to care for the chronic and persistent wounds of war. This model of care persists today in what are called State Veteran Homes (SVH). These chronic care facilities provide institutionalized care to more than sixteen thousand military Veterans across the nation. These facilities are constructed with joint funding of the state and federal government with federal dollars provided through the VHA. Ongoing care is provided by state employees or contractors engaged by the states, but the cost of these personnel is substantially funded by the VHA. An advantage of these facilities is the ability to also admit a Veteran's spouse who needs care and desires to be with his or her Veteran, something precluded by federal law in a VHA-owned and operated facility.

The VHA assures the quality of care delivered in these state-owned and operated facilities through biannual inspections conducted by VHA employees or geriatric experts under contract to the VHA. However, the law enabling these inspections is very clear that the VHA has no operational role in correcting problems identified during those inspections. The only outcome of a failed inspection is to report the finding to the state and, if not corrected the VHA, may bar payment for or stop future Veteran admissions. This course of action, in turn, has the potential to harm the Veteran and not the state. To my knowledge, the bar to future admissions has never been used to enforce performance or quality improvement of these state-owned facilities.

There is, unfortunately, no standardized model or enabling law that assures these state-owned facilities are managed professionally. Geriatric care of individual patients continues to emerge in American health care with substantial complexity. The professional management or, more accurately stated, the failure to deliver professional management to these facilities resulted in some horrific outcomes during the pandemic. In some states, the operation of these facilities is assigned to a state official who then contracts for an outside management service to deliver care to a state's Veterans. Budgets are determined by the amount of federal per diem payment for each Veteran and then supplemented by a state revenue stream. It is common for individual states to have no in-house geriatric or institutional elder care expertise within the state-based oversight offices, so they often don't even know what to look for as they provide oversight.

As the pandemic progressed, the VHA began to recognize the vulnerability of the entire Veteran population over the age of sixty-five years. We also recognized that the pressure in some states for acute care beds was resulting in the transfer of patients to long-term care facilities who were not ready to accept these transfers safely. These transfers could only be accomplished safely if the facilities followed the complex COVID-19 positive and negative infection control policies that have been discussed previously. We began to hear of problems in multiple state-run facilities, especially in New Jersey, whose facilities were under the control of the adjutant general of the New Jersey National Guard. This structure of leadership provided little or no geriatric care expertise. These management, staffing, and professional training shortcomings highlighted multiple failures to protect the most vulnerable of the institutionalized elder population.

The failure to understand how to protect this population of patients is based primarily on the need to isolate employees actively working with COVID-19-positive patients from those working in COVID-19-negative patient rooms, as has been discussed previously. The effective isolation of the positive and negative neighborhoods within a facility was complicated by locally generated directives that even precluded health care personnel from wearing gloves and masks. State officials in New Jersey generated these directives in an apparent effort to avoid alarming residents. The spread of the virus was further facilitated by continued use of congregate dining rooms for patients, which brought large numbers of infected patients and staff into contact with uninfected patients. With professional nursing staffing very low, compounded by the absence of trained infection control personnel, the ability to institute effective infection control protocols was thus impossible.

This resulted in about one hundred and nineteen Veteran deaths in the state of New Jersey alone. [37] The same type of events occurred in SVHs across the nation. Although exact numbers are unavailable, it is estimated that COVID-19 Veteran deaths exceeded 1145 across 110 SVHs, with death rates in state-run homes doubling what was experienced in VHA long-term care facilities. There were 110 deaths in a western New York facility, sixty-two in a single facility located in the southern tip of Maryland, forty-seven in Wisconsin, and forty-four in Ohio. One of the most egregious examples of the inability to control infections occurred at the Yukio Okutsu State Veterans Home in Hawaii, where twenty-seven Veterans died of COVID-19 in the fall of 2020. The facility was managed during this time by an outside contractor based in Utah. [38] In all of these deaths, the operational failure was the same: an inability to control infection spread until the number of deaths completely overwhelmed the facility. These examples are a perfect reflection of my earlier reference to finding subject matter experts and deferring to their expertise. In all of these cases, no experts in infection control or elder care were even engaged.

In each of these states and many others, the VHA eventually provided professional nursing and geriatric expertise as well as infection control personnel at the request of state governors to train state or contract employees in effective infection control and prevention and the use of personal protective measures. Those VHA teams remained sometimes for many weeks in active contact with state Veteran care leaders. Unfortunately, these deaths reflected exactly the same problems seen in commercial (non-Veteran) extended care facilities across the nation.

By November 2020, the Kaiser Family Foundation (KFF) would report that more than 100,000 patients in long-term care facilities across the United States had died of COVID-19. This was 40 percent of the total COVID-19 deaths in the United States at that time. The KFF released the following statement: "And it raises questions about whether nursing homes and other facilities are able to protect their residents and, if not, what actions can be taken to mitigate the threat posed by the virus."

To attempt to quantify the enormity of this problem, there are 65,600 long-term care facilities (LTC) in the United States. These facilities provide about one million LTC beds. It is estimated that as many as 70 percent of aging Americans will need some type of long-term care over their lifetimes. In 2016, the most recent data available states that 8.3 million Americans received care in one of these facilities (National Center for Health Statistics, 2019). [39]

The VHA model of professional nursing centric care, supported by experienced specialists in infection control and geriatrics previously outlined, and the creation of COVID-19-positive and negative neighborhoods protected Veterans in VHA-managed extended care facilities. The validity of that protection was reflected in COVID-19 patient death rates that were one-half of the commercial and State Veteran Home LTC facility rates across the nation. [40] The nation, as it evaluates how the most at-risk institutionalized patients fared during this pandemic, must fundamentally reexamine the model of elder care currently available to the vast majority of non-service-disabled Veterans. The failure to include extended or long-term care coverage under the current Medicare benefit package forces the cost burden for this care upon a small subset of patients and their families able to sustain the cost of this care for their loved ones. This results in the need to minimize the use of professional nurses in order to control costs. The result is an unprepared workforce composed primarily of nursing assistants without the benefit of continuously available facility-based trained personnel able to immediately support and mitigate the effects of a public health emergency such as this.

In 2021, Genworth (a longtime dominant player in the US long-term care insurance market) completed a cost-of-care survey in the United States and demonstrated that monthly facility-based "skilled" extended (or long-term) care approached almost $9,000 per month or almost $110,000 a year for a private room. A semiprivate extended care room lowered that cost by about $1,000 per month. Extended care facilities are designated at their lowest level as assisted living. Facilities designated at this level thus provide the lowest level of patient assistance. Care levels then graduate upward to what is termed nursing homes and then to nursing homes with a "skilled" designator to indicate higher levels of care provision. The difference in professional nursing staffing between commercial care facilities designated as assisted living, nursing homes, and skilled nursing homes is less significant than might be anticipated and varies from state to state based on the nuances of state licensure. CMS (Centers for Medicare and Medicaid Services) mandates that there be licensed professional RN staffing for at least eight hours of each day in a facility designated as skilled and that at least 30 percent of staffed employee hours be from an

RN. This level of professional nursing is degraded as one moves downward from skilled to basic nursing home to assisted living facilities. [41]

As the population of the United States over the age of sixty-five approaches 20 percent, the need for these facilities is ever-increasing. As the burden of twenty-four-hour care for some elder patients exceeds the ability of home-based and family-delivered care to render a safe and effective environment, the nation must grapple with facility-based care that is escalating in cost each year. [42] In addition, the need to create care models that acknowledge the ever-increasing demand for nurses and the failure of nursing education programs to supply nurses in adequate numbers to deliver care to this expanding patient population is increasing rapidly. In addition, the current nursing practice theory that defines the current model of bedside nursing for these patients must be reexamined. Finally, the escalation of nursing pay rates during the pandemic has highlighted the impending shortage of these essential, skilled bedside caregivers. A potential solution that acknowledges these patients' needs for a comprehensive care team under the direction of a professional nurse can include certified nursing assistants, but there must be enough patient and professional nurse interaction each day to ensure care safety.

Within the military care system, combat medics are used in support of this category of patients' needs and are actively supported by a team that includes professional nurses. This care team model in military acute care facilities is a proven model of successful care that should be examined as a potential model of care extension in civilian long-term care facilities. This recommended reexamination should include raising the skill competencies of the CNA and the development of specially trained geriatric care paramedics for potential use in long-term care settings.

The costs of these new models of care delivery should incorporate the development of enhanced ability for the delivery of care in the patient's home. Home-based care should provide robust professional support and care integration that directly reduces the burden of care provision by family members in the home. Recognition of the ultimate savings to society as well as the enhanced physical and mental wellbeing of patients remaining in their homes must be quantified. When needed, traditional facility-based care must recognize the lessons of the COVID-19 pandemic, and federal regulations must then evolve in order to guarantee safe staffing of care teams for the nation's most vulnerable.

Finally, the lessons of the New Jersey, Hawaii, and multiple other SVHs should include changing VHA oversight regulations to include the ability for VHA to immediately assume operational control of state-run Veteran homes following failed inspections in order to rapidly assure the safety of Veterans housed in those facilities for care. This should apply in times of emergency and chronic failure to meet inspection standards.

CHAPTER FIFTEEN

Joining the Military

"God gives me the stability of today to be ready for the chaos of tomorrow."

THIS IS A PRINCIPLE that I have followed for most of my life. I have discussed earlier the family and personal turmoil that existed early in my life as our family was torn by parental alcoholism and spousal physical abuse. This is a quote that I have used for years paraphrasing several biblical references that capture life as I know it. It was introduced to me as a teenager by a Methodist minister who was a friend of our family as we discussed faith and our responsibility as individuals to our society and world over a combined family dinner. It became part of my leadership philosophy on December 1, 1969.

I recognized how close chaos was to each of our lives when my own life as an uninformed, unaware, and unencumbered college student was startled back to reality on the evening of December 1, 1969. I was a freshman in college at Western Michigan University in Kalamazoo, Michigan, when America conducted its first draft lottery since the 1942 conscription of ten million soldiers in order to create the Army that would eventually win WWII.

This current lottery would be conducted in order to prioritize each of us as potential military draftees available for the Vietnam War. A large glass bowl was placed on a table in the selective service offices in Washington, DC. It held within the bowl 366 blue plastic balls with every possible birthdate printed on each of them. The selected birthdates would be applied to those men between age eighteen and twenty-six years old at the time of the drawing. The drawing of the balls from the glass bowl was televised. Notification for call-up to service, it had been announced, would begin in January 1970 and continue for the first half of 1970 for those who would turn nineteen years old during the calendar year (I turned nineteen in April 1970). The selective service, for which we were obligated to register when we had turned eighteen, had announced that each month, thirty numbers would be called for their military entrance physicals starting in January 1970. In February 1970, numbers thirty-one through sixty would be called, and so on each month through the first six months of the year 1970. For those who had their physicals in January, induction for those categorized as "1-A" after their physical was May 1970. Chaos and a severe dose of reality was about to enter each of our lives on that 1st of December.

I was a high school competitive wrestler whose primary goal in college was to earn a place on the college wrestling team. When I graduated from high school, my grades reflected my dedication to success in sports not academics. I had trained daily since high school graduation to be selected for what, at that time, was a very good WMU wrestling team. I was what is termed a "walk on" athlete without scholarship. Since I had arrived at the university in August, my entire focus was on sports and training to compete at the NCAA Division One college level. Vietnam and the draft were far away from what I was thinking about. Most nights, however, at dinner in the dormitory cafeteria, discussion of the war and the draft occurred.

It was 1969, and student antiwar activists and protestors distributed leaflets as we ate dinner, inviting us to antiwar protests to be conducted initially on Saturdays as protesting students stopped traffic, carried signs, and chanted slogans on campus. Many of these activists walked around at dinner, talking earnestly to each of us about how to protect ourselves from tear gas should the "pigs" use it on us during the protest. It was noisy and chaotic as I walked across campus to the fieldhouse to train on Saturdays that fall. Soon the chaos of these protests would overwhelm the university nearly every day.

Across America, most campuses and their students would learn the smell and burn of tear gas as it wafted across the universities. I would personally feel the fear as I watched the Michigan State Police clear the roadway in the center of my campus of protestors as they tapped their night sticks against their riot shields with each step forward that they took.

I didn't understand any of it. Nor did I think I should "work to get out of the draft," as they suggested. I was, after all, completely healthy without any of the health problems or "weak ankles" that many of my fellow college students believed would preclude their individual selection as a fully healthy 1-A candidate for military service. What would cause a military entrance physician to identify you as less than 1-A and, therefore, not fit for military duty was the topic many of my friends were discussing while at meals in the cafeteria. The maladies each of them discussed with significant conviction they believed would cause them to fail the military entrance physical.

A number of my high school graduation classmates and friends had already completed these physicals after graduation. In southeastern Michigan, where I graduated from high school, about 60 percent of my high school class went directly to the auto manufacturing plants out of high school, just as their parents had. Most had never considered college, and their future was clear: a lifetime of work building cars that would guarantee their livelihoods for life. For most of them, the draft was a delay to their entrance to a good life that most of their parents and even grandparents had led with the United Auto Workers union and Ford, Chrysler, or General Motors.

For all of us at the university, however, the war in Southeast Asia seemed so far away until that night of December 1st. On that night, all of our lives could change regardless of what position our birthday was chosen. I, like many of my classmates, had taken time away from school over the few weeks preceding December 1st to visit Army, Navy, and Air Force recruiting stations in order to discuss my options with recruiters. The conversation centered on if I should enlist rather than wait for the draft. Each of the recruiters had sincerely explained why joining the military before the draft lottery was essential to my being accepted into the branch of the service I desired. But I didn't desire any of them at that time. Nevertheless, I had the paperwork for enlistment into each branch of the service on my lap as I sat on the floor in my dorm room watching the small television, we were lucky enough to have. The paperwork was stacked with the "contract" with the Air Force on the top of the pile.

I threw a blanket on the floor of my dorm room, and I watched the selection of dates with at least ten additional eighteen- to twenty-one-year-old men packed into the room on chairs, the beds, and the floor. We were all loud and boisterous and full of bravado until the first ball was chosen.

It then became deathly quiet. All across the hallways and individual rooms of this giant all male dormitory, there was quiet as a congressman from the House Armed Services Committee reached into the bowl and chose the first ball. "September 14th." Everyone had left the doors to the hallway open, and from across the hall, someone yelled, "Shit!" Suddenly, there was movement across the hall where a similar group had gathered. The student who had spoken now walked out of the room alone with his head down and went down the emergency stairs to the outside. I didn't know him except as one of the guys across the hall.

My birthday is April 25th. The second number pulled from the glass bowl was April 24th. I couldn't breathe as the month "April" and then the number "twenty . . ." was spoken. As the word "fourth" was added, I could breathe again. It was like a weight was removed from my chest. We all paused for any verbal outburst or motion from those in the room and adjoining rooms, but there was none. My birthday, April 25th, would eventually be chosen 252nd. I was safe, but the chaos of the war had changed each of our lives and communities.

Within two days, the September 14th birthday student across the hall had joined the Marines. He left school immediately following announcing his decision to join as there was "no reason to finish the semester." In 1970, the highest number eventually drafted was 195, September 24th. I was safe. I avoided chaos by the luck of the draw.

I found the entire process completely unfair and in no way felt good about being 252nd. I decided over Christmas break that I would join the Navy and announced this to my parents by telephone after my return to the university in January 1970.

I told them I intended to finish my first year of college and join in the spring of 1970. My dad, I'm sure at my mom's insistence, immediately drove from southeastern Michigan to Kalamazoo to talk to me about the decision.

He arrived calm and thoughtful, as always. He let me talk first while introducing the fact that my mom was pretty upset with this decision. I discussed with him my feeling of profound regret that frankly had surprised me after the lottery. It was the exact same feeling of loss that overwhelmed me when we moved away from Mt. Clemens (and the Safety Patrol) many years previously. Dad listened intently and discussed the responsibility each of us have in serving our communities and nation. He discussed the responsibilities of citizenship and helping others that he felt motivated my decision to serve. He then shared for the first time a number of experiences in his life, including his service to the nation as a public health service officer during and after WWII. Because of his expertise in infectious disease, he was drafted into the Army and placed in the public health service.

I was a freshman pre-medicine student at the time of the lottery, and after more than an hour of talking, he asked that I consider delaying entrance to the military until I could serve as a doctor as he had. He also asked that we discuss this over the upcoming summer since I wanted to finish the school year we had already paid for. I hesitantly agreed, but the feeling that I had unfairly avoided military service continued for many years. I would leave my wrestling career at the end of the first year as it no longer seemed that important to me as I concentrated on studying to become the best physician I could be. In the spring of 1971, I was told by one of my roommates that the

"September 14th" guy across the hall was killed in Vietnam. I never knew his name.

In the days after being told of his death, my decision to join the military and serve the nation had become unwavering. Life and prolonged years of medical training would delay my entrance to uniformed service. The feelings of regret would revisit me as America became engaged in Operation Desert Storm in 1990, and I realized that the decision to serve had never changed.

On April 24, 1991, I finally was commissioned in the Army Reserve. Every day since, the quote from so many years previously has been an enduring and unwavering principle of my work. Utilize the calm of today to prepare for the chaos of tomorrow. I will never forget my feeling of intense debt that the calm I experienced to train and learn my profession was protected and guaranteed by those whose "numbers" were called before mine—my work since is made possible by what they did and the sacrifices that they made. We each have an option in life to prepare for the inevitability of life's chaos or ignore its inevitability and react after it occurs. I prefer the former.

CHAPTER SIXTEEN

Preparing For Chaos

ALL OF US WHO have faced a serious health-related personal challenge wish we had physically exercised just a little more or eaten in a healthier manner. This is especially true when an unforeseen health problem falls unexpectedly upon us. But what I am about to describe is organizational and not personal preparation.

From an organizational standpoint, a willingness to invest in readiness for the inconceivable or impossible event is a delicate balance with daily operational demands. There are always those who will criticize the investment in materials or training for the rare or inconceivable event. Dr. Kadlec as the ASPR was criticized for investing in bioterror preparations to reduce risk if such an attack should occur. He was criticized even as the pandemic occurred (instead of a bioterrorism attack), as if the nation could have had more supplies for use against the COVID-19 specific threat.

Hindsight is easy for those not charged with attempting to "see" the future. This pandemic has taught all of us who were accountable leaders during this time significant, humbling, and difficult lessons. This is part of the reason I wanted to write this book. There are stories to be told and lessons to be learned and acted upon, but no one should attempt to predict the future or prepare for only one thing. Instead, we must prepare our teams and organizations to be agile, resilient, and aware of what we are likely and unlikely to face and think through who and what we will need to do in response. Crisis planning can become all-consuming, but leaders must balance this preparation for the inconceivable with managing the day-to-day challenges of their organizations to be ready for anything, even on a sunny day when life seems routine and calm. Consider the story I related of mass casualties generated in the German bus bombing. We thought we were ready, but cultural differences between the allied forces disrupted our response.

This pandemic has taught us that command and control of this nation's emergency operational health response system must be robustly developed and elevated in stature. Improvements to emergency health response operations and planning needs to be codified into law or federal regulation. Let me provide an example of how I view this challenge from the national defense structure. The United States protects itself and its people from external threats through the National Security Council (NSC), which is the president's principal forum for the consideration of national security and foreign policy matters. The NSC receives advice from the uniformed chairman of the Joint Chiefs of Staff, who, while the senior most military officer of our nation, commands no troops but instead serves as the principal military advisor to the president. The NSC formalizes at the most senior levels of the executive branch, under the direction of the president of the United States, the tools to protect the nation from identified or even as yet unidentified threats.

This pandemic has revealed that global public health threats deserve the same level of senior White House engagement. The

NSC was authorized under the National Security Act of 1947 following WWII and was reorganized in the Executive Office of the President in 1949. It has been tested and matured in its functions since that time. By contrast, there is no unifying medical structure that mimics or even internally supports the NSC with operational medical expertise. (There are excellent public health, subject matter experts on the NSC but not experts in operational health care delivery.)

Unlike many of our allies, America does not have a unified national health system, but I would ask that the reader not immediately assume that I am arguing for the creation of a government-owned unified national health system. The vast majority of the available health delivery assets across the United States are privately owned and with the existence of a smaller but no less essential DOD, VA and IHS (Indian Health Service) government-operated systems. The pandemic has revealed that there needs to be an overarching command and control mechanism that ensures the stability of American citizens' ability to access care in a crisis. This requirement will need an NSC-like structure within the Executive Office of the President for future pandemic or public health responses. The use of the vice-president conducting a daily gathering of an ad hoc committee convened during the early stages of this pandemic reflects the lack of an effective national public health emergency response structure. The development of this capability would also ensure that the voice of health system operations is clearly heard by the most senior government leaders before decisions on the distribution of crisis response capabilities are made. Although there are public health bodies like CDC and HHS with a clear voice in planning and policy there is no operational health care delivery coordinating body for federal health response. Congress should consider this shortfall for correction immediately.

There are, in preparation for disasters, enumerated Emergency Support Functions (ESF) in the US government federal disaster response system. These functions are coordinated by FEMA. These functions are numbered, and the medical response is contained within what is referred to as ESF 8, with HHS identified as the responsible agency. The ESF 8 Annex, which covers this area of federal response, acknowledges the private sector "leadership" role in health emergencies and concentrates its guidance on support for logistics, movement of patients, and mortuary affairs. What ESF 8 does not effectively do is create an interface for coordinating this envisioned command and control "leadership" to manage casualties that outstrip the capacity of a regional health care delivery system. The American people remain at risk until this capability is defined, developed, tested, and sustained.

Readiness for war is a difficult concept to attain when applied to trauma and surgery-related health care. Maintenance of individual skills for a trauma surgeon requires significant volumes of patients that have sustained injuries similar to combat. The ability to then deliver to deployed locations around the world critical numbers of these personnel with trauma specialist expertise from those sustainment training sites has substantial and very complex operational implications. Those implications include how to sustain services in the facility that deploys the trauma-skilled provider to the crisis, and therefore no longer has the capacity to deliver care. For example, the United States has a significant shortage of neurosurgeons. This is a problem in virtually every American health care system, private or government owned. The removal of neurosurgeons or trauma surgeons from a military hospital or a civilian hospital where a surgeon may be actively providing patient care while serving in the reserve components of the military will create a deficit in the ability to deliver care to those institutions that are losing the SME (neurosurgeon). The primary rationale for leaving those surgeons in their current location is the sustainment of combat readiness that is dependent on the surgeon's ability to sustain individual surgical skills. This skill readiness is maintained by completing surgeries on patients using the most modern equipment and medical techniques available. A surgeon needed for the rare and unpredictable episodes of combat casualty care simply cannot sit idle for months, waiting for patients while their skills degrade. This would create a potentially unsafe situation for potential wartime casualties.

DOD's ability to sustain both wartime readiness and conduct a robust domestic health care response capability was encumbered by what I have previously referred to as a large number of "in an abundance of caution" domestic deployments where there were few patients in need of care. Recognizing these issues in mission assignment, the role of the VHA to serve as a backstop to the American health care system should be formalized and balanced with demands on DOD. This balance should include more explicitly defining VHA's role in regional bed management and the domestic response as part of ESF 8 under HHS command and control.

Only through clearly defining this balance of responsibilities between each large federal delivery system can each department effectively grow domestic capabilities, including the sustainment of dedicated civilian mobile response assets. This also creates the opportunity to coordinate the combined usage of materials in both VA and DOD-assigned missions.

The command and control of this response should recognize existing DOD and VHA medical command and control capability and the recommended creation of the ability to communicate on a common domestic crisis communication system with civilian-supported community health facilities. This already-reviewed communication problem is an additional structural weakness that should be corrected.

CHAPTER SEVENTEEN

Innovation

HEALTH CARE CRISIS RESPONSE requires the ability of leaders engaged in the response to innovate. I have discussed previously the role rapid decision-making makes in ensuring success and allowing operational decisions to be made, even when all information is not available. We have defined this previously as "the 60-percent rule." In addition to agile and rapid decision-making, however, the ability to support innovation requires an environment that acknowledges the need to innovate even in material supply when faced with unique challenges. This acknowledgment should include recognition that those operating as innovators within health systems engage in a risky endeavor and oftentimes experience failure.

An example of this crisis response innovation occurred while I was deployed to Afghanistan in late 2003. An elementary school had been bombed by the Taliban, causing a large number of pediatric casualties, challenging our blood supply as already discussed. An American military combat hospital is generally deployed with equipment to care for diseases and trauma to service members who are, by and large, healthy young adults. The US military combat trauma hospital is not staffed, nor is it equipped for pediatric trauma or pediatric critical care.

Ventilators, IV pumps, and anesthesia machines are designed and fielded for anticipated use in young adults. Service members also have few comorbid conditions and, prior to injury, are in very good physical condition.

Following the bombing of the elementary school, the Bagram-based US Army combat hospital received about two dozen catastrophically injured children under the age of eleven in the few hours following the bombing. The trauma teams from the US would perform more than a dozen limb amputations on these children because of massive blast injuries. In addition, most would need ventilator care for blast-related pulmonary injuries. A pediatric ventilator has different pressure and rate settings than an adult ventilator, and ventilator circuits (tubing) are also different than an adult ventilator. The purpose of these machines is to "breathe" oxygen into and carbon dioxide out of the child whose lungs cannot do the work of breathing without mechanical support. Unfortunately, no pediatric ventilator circuits were available to the US military medical team as the children began arriving.

The ability to reduce the total volume of air moved into and out of the lungs of a small child is defined as a "circuit." These tubes provide appropriate pressure, resistance, and volume of air to the patient. Each of these are essential variables in effective pediatric vs. adult airway management. As we recognized the potential for massive pediatric death due to the absence of these circuits, the ICU nurses, respiratory therapists, and the nurse and physician anesthesia providers quickly redesigned adult ventilator circuits in order to care for these children. Their innovation saved almost all of these children until we could obtain ventilators designed for pediatric patients. It is notable that in 2003, almost none of this technology was available in any civilian Afghan hospital. If these children were not cared for by the American military hospital, they would have almost certainly all perished. The innovation provided by these soldiers went well beyond their expected mission.

VHA provides substantial research to advance the understanding of diseases and injuries sustained by Veterans in their service to the nation. VHA had established an office of innovation led by two remarkable clinicians, Dr. Ryan Vega and Dr. Beth Ripley, when 3D printing or additive manufacturing capability was first imagined. This innovation infrastructure would unexpectedly become an essential component of our COVID-19 response. The ability to provide agile advanced manufacturing, bioprinting of live cells, and the ability to complete surgical planning was all facilitated by the availability of 3D printing under the direction of these leaders. These tools allowed surgeons to hold a 3D printed model of a tumor and its collocated organs and vascular structures in their hands prior to actual surgery. These tools had already (prior to COVID-19) reduced actual surgical time and reduced patient risk from complex surgeries.

As the nation began to experience shortages of consumable medical materials as the volume of COVID-19 patients increased, VHA funded the robust expansion of our 3D printing capability across the nation. The inability to obtain even the cotton swabs used to obtain COVID-19 nasal samples was accelerating across the nation. We found that we could create the fluid (what the laboratory industry refers to as "media") to transport COVID-19 tests but could not obtain the nasal swabs that were inserted into patient's noses as we collected specimens for COVID-19 testing. In addition, high-risk procedures like intubation (inserting a tube into a patient's lungs) and CPR created significant viral particle spread in patient rooms that even fitted N95 masks did not sufficiently protect VHA staff from virus exposure. Personnel in these situations wear positive air pressure respirators (PAPR) that protect them. These PAPR hoods were also unavailable anywhere in the nation as the pandemic accelerated. Doctors Vega and Ripley began 3D printing key PAPR hood parts and entered into a partnership with American private sector industry to manufacture all the PAPR hoods and the nasal swabs VHA would need for our pandemic response.

3D printing is also referred to as additive manufacturing that allows for the construction of three-dimensional objects under computer control. In this manufacturing process, materials are deposited, joined, and solidified layer by layer. Actual limited available parts of PAPRs and nasal swabs were created all over the nation through the use of these VHA owned printers. They prevented VHA from exhausting our supply of these materials and reduced our demand on a limited commercial supply chain.

Sustainment of this type of innovation requires funds and must acknowledge that inventors and innovators are not always successful. Tolerance of failure includes the recognition that sometimes resources are not effectively consumed and linked to an ultimate value. This fact required substantial effort on the part of senior VA leaders who demonstrated, even at the VA secretary level, a fundamental understanding of this work. This was another example where the CARES Act provided funds to enable this work to continue and be ultimately successful.

VHA found itself with multiple types of 3D printing technology across the nation. Ongoing work to fully leverage the capacity of these tools will reveal a substantial future value beyond what has already been discussed. The support of the Food and Drug Administration, who acted in full partnership with VHA, substantially facilitated VHA's development of additive manufactured products, such as the PAPR, and was a testament to the long-standing relationships between FDA and the VHA's Center for Innovation. Both agencies advanced significantly by utilization of the partnership initiated well before the pandemic.

The shortage of these materials brings us to one of the most difficult operational challenges of the pandemic: the sustainment of the American medical supply chain. There are two major divisions of the medical supply chain for the sake of this discussion. The first is the non-consumable items, such as ventilators, bedside monitoring devices, and even hospital beds. The second is the consumable supplies, such as the items included in personal protective equipment. Examples of these include various types of masks, gloves, gowns, foot covering, hoods, eye protection, and so on.

Many tasks in a hospital require both—a non-consumable core machine with consumable pieces that are replaced for each patient. Because of this, the sustainability of non-consumable items are often dependent on consumables to sustain function. The best example of this was discussed in the previous chapter regarding the pediatric ventilators in Afghanistan. A non-consumable ventilator is attached to consumable plastic tubing called a "circuit" that is ultimately disposed of after the patient no longer needs the tubing in order to breathe.

Non-consumable supplies are usually purchased on an intermittent or occasional basis, and few if any of those supplies are kept in hospital warehouses. Although only 25 percent of ventilators may be in use at any given time in a hospital, the remaining are readily available in ICU rooms not in use or in collocated storage facilities near the ICU. Rarely would a ventilator be used in a non-ICU hospital room except in specialty rooms designated for chronic ventilator dependent patients. As the pandemic began and the New York governor predicted the need for tens of thousands of ventilators, the VHA began assessing our own possible ventilator need. About this time, Deb Kramer returned to VHA from a temporary role in the VA Office of Whistle Blower Protection, where she had worked to ensure the protection of whistleblowers after the 2014 access to care crisis. Her return to logistics management reflected her skill as an experienced Army medical logistician whose talent would ultimately sustain us as we faced the impending and ever-emerging challenges of supply and logistics during the pandemic.

Deb is a former US Army Medical Service Corps officer with extensive deployment experience as a combat medic, operating room technician and eventually as an acquisition officer. She has a master of science degree in biotechnology and had been working in multiple roles across the VA since 2012. Her appointment as the acting assistant under secretary for health for support services early in the pandemic reflected our need for a consummate professional to lead this area.

As the governor of New York asked for ventilators, it appeared that all ventilators in the national strategic stockpile were likely going to be distributed very early in the pandemic, leaving few if any for emerging needs elsewhere. Acquisition of this type of material by the US government usually requires competitive bidding between vendors that can take many months to complete to ensure the best value for the agency (and the American taxpayer). This acquisition process would include the development of a formal requirements document, conversion of those requirements to a government-approved request for proposal, solicitation of vendors that includes review of potential preference for the use of service-disabled small business suppliers, assessment of vendor proposals by a board of experts, and final award by a government contracting official. This process can take a year or more in development and execution before an award is completed. The initial material delivery can then be dependent upon available manufacturing capability and material availability.

Clearly, this entire model of acquisition was unacceptably slow in a crisis, but fortunately, Deb Kramer and her team were able to move the agency to what is called "directed" (expedited and directed to a single vendor) awards. She was instrumental in understanding the crisis and legal ramifications of bypassing a complex acquisition system that was ill-prepared for this type of rapid response. I should add that the support of several VA attorneys who were experts in acquisition law was essential to executing this rapid procurement of materials quickly but legally.

The presence of robust funding from the CARES Act would again become essential to the ability of VHA to compete with commercial healthcare delivery systems in an acquisition process that would, in many cases, escalate cost by three to ten times the normal cost for a non-consumable item. VHA logistics and acquisitions, under Deb's leadership, demonstrated the ability to secure the consumable materials that were part of a ventilator circuit (as discussed in the previous combat example) and millions of other items. This was essential to the rapid fielding of these materials as VHA purchased and fielded to medical centers thousands of ventilators, thousands of hospital beds, and the associated monitors as we expanded our acute care footprint over a matter of weeks. The consumption rate of appropriated dollars accelerated as well as the presence of predatory vendors who now demanded payment in advance for many of these materials.

Payment in advance is not allowed in federal government material acquisition, and demand for this type of payment created significant challenges as we competed across a landscape where hundreds of government acquisition officers were on the telephone and internet continuously trying to buy materials that were sold while they discussed with the seller the government's inability to prepay. This limited our suppliers to long-term government vendors who were financially stable and recognized that vendor and customer relationships must be sustained long term. Despite this, many of the executed contracts failed to deliver the required products due to a myriad of supply chain and competitive challenges disrupted by COVID-19 as every hospital and vendor in the world began to buy up what they could. This forced the requirement for significant redistribution of materials following delivery to an individual medical center. As redistribution of materials occurred between care delivery locations, VHA began to recognize the need for an internal regional distribution platform that spanned the entirety of our network.

VHA purchases huge volumes of consumable supplies similar to most major health care and even retail delivery systems. As consumable materials such as bandages are utilized, there is a message sent from an individual nursing care unit to a medical center warehouse or logistics office to trigger the resupply of those materials. This might occur in the consuming ICU, operating room, or a nursing unit within an individual hospital.

Well-run, large enterprises such as VHA run this type of program within what is called a "just in time" delivery model. This means that a vendor truck arrives at the hospital just about the time the last package of bandages is opened. This avoids having large amounts of materials sitting on shelves and avoids the possibility that time-sensitive items like pharmaceuticals could expire while waiting to be used. In this type of just-in-time system, there needs to be a stable demand signal or better stated, the amount of material consumed is very predictable. This allows the supplying vendor and the medical center logistics system to reliably predict usage and appropriate stockage levels to prevent exhaustion of supply for any item. In a large hospital, this system would apply to as many as 10,000 separate consumable items.

In VHA, there are ongoing contracts with large commercial vendors around the country to supply thousands of these consumable supplies. In addition, there is more than one vendor in each area to ensure reliability and redundancy. These supplies are visible on software programs that also predict the delivery dates of materials and can adjust for increasing or decreasing demand of a certain item in an individual facility. In most cases, a logistician can "see" a delivery of material as much as six weeks out.

Most of these consumable materials are discarded after a single patient use. It should be noted that there is no evidence that this concept of disposal of a protective mask after one patient per use actually protects the patient or employee any better than a staff member wearing an unsoiled and undamaged mask for an entire day of patient care (or even longer). In operating a system as large as the VHA, there could be the consumption of more than 250 thousand face masks by nursing care personnel each day and more than one million gloves daily, even prior to the pandemic. Because the VHA has an emergency operations mission, actual supplies of these materials on hand at VHA locations often exceeded ninety days of predicted routine levels of usage at the start of the pandemic.

As the pandemic began to spread across the world, several unstable process risks were identified. First, almost all these consumable materials are not manufactured in the United States. The vast majority are from Southeast Asia and China. It is likely obvious to the reader that when there is worldwide pressure for materials, nations will protect their own people before they sell to foreign nations, and this applies even to America's allies. We began, at this point, to recognize that delivery times for our US-based prime vendors (almost always, these vendors were intermediaries, not the actual manufacturers) were increasing significantly in time from ordering to actual material delivery. We also recognized that visibility of those orders were no longer showing in our software systems. I ask the reader to think about what happens when you or I am ordering a product on Amazon, and the Amazon software system identifies that there are limited quantities available. You or I might order quickly and in greater quantity than we need so we don't run out of whatever we are ordering. (Think of paper good shortages.) Medical material acquisition officers across the world began to order extras to ensure they didn't run out of a needed item. When this occurs across the entire nation or the entire world, the supply system collapses.

Substantial media attention was directed at health care system supplies as smaller health delivery systems were unable to compete with large systems to keep adequate supplies on hand. You may remember images or stories of doctors and nurses wearing black trash bags instead of gowns, for example. This led to several directives on emergency use of these materials by the CDC. Media headlines would portray this collapse of the system as follows:

> *"How the world ran out of everything" – New York Times, Oct 22, 2021* [43]

At the same time, there was also rapid depletion of materials from prime vendor warehouses. This depletion occurred at the same time as the government began discussing the problem of hoarding of materials in conjunction with the possible use of what is called the Defense Production Act (DPA). The DPA is a law that was passed in 1950 to ensure appropriate war material was available for mobilization for the Korean war. The act requires businesses to accept and prioritize government contracts for materials necessary for national defense. It also gives the president certain powers to combat price gouging and hoarding. The act further outlines criminal penalties for violation of the act and provides the president some control over the civilian economy.

As the strategic national stockpile was rapidly approaching depletion, there was broad recognition across health system providers of the lack of domestic production capacity for most of these materials. Senior leaders began to discuss the president's potential use of his authorities under the Defense Production Act, but no vendor had experienced the implementation of this law in seventy years. We also discovered that, as written in the DPA, VHA was not specifically called out for priority delivery of materials and is lumped together with all other health system providers. At this point in time, our long-term supplier relationships evaporated almost overnight as those suppliers attempted to prepare to meet the requirements of the impending implementation of the DPA. The entire medical supply chain quickly became unstable as the consumption rates continued to skyrocket. In addition, the visibility of possible future deliveries was completely wiped out just as suddenly.

As VHA acquisition experts could no longer see incoming shipments, they contacted their prime vendors, who stated that they were waiting for directions from government leaders to see if they could continue to fill their contractually required materials or would these materials fall under the DPA requirements and be sent elsewhere. In response, the VHA's supplies inventory continued to rapidly degrade in numbers and availability.

VHA began rebalancing materials to areas of acute shortages across the regions but also decided that we must attempt to reduce daily consumption as much as possible. If we failed, we would be unable to protect anyone, and the system would collapse. We instituted, at my direction, "crisis directives" to reduce the consumption of masks. We did this to avoid letting the enterprise move below a fourteen-day supply of masks (the reader should remember we began with an excess of a ninety-day supply). Employees in contact with patients would be given priority for the most protective (N95), masks and those with little or no risk of patient contact would wear surgical masks rather than the N95 (personally fitted) mask. These would be worn for an entire day of work unless contaminated or damaged. This decision reduced the consumption of materials but substantially challenged the long-held culture of mask disposal after every patient. It also increased employee fear as events were occurring so quickly that there was little warning to employees that this decision was even being considered. As a senior leader who still provides bedside patient care, I understood the fear that these decisions created in our heroic workforce. Unfortunately, there were no other choices to be made. Either reduce the consumption of materials or reduce our availability to provide care for patients. The latter was not acceptable and would violate our commitment to the American people.

Although web-based training for mask usage under the emergency use guidelines was released, the erosion of employee and management trust from this decision would take many weeks to be restored. I recorded multiple daily employee videos regarding the decision. These were released directly to all employees, and they elicited a significant response to my email inbox. We attempted to respond to every one of those emails in an effort to restore as much transparency as possible.

There is no greater responsibility for any leader than to protect the safety of their workforce. I have been in situations over my career where I wondered if my leader understood the challenges, I was facing on the front line of patient care. Many of the email communications I received during this time questioned my commitment to employee safety. We worked continuously to restore what I believed was eroded trust as the world grappled with an unprecedented shortage of these materials.

Throughout this time, Deb Kramer's team searched the world for PPE and purchased materials as quickly as was possible under the various emergency purchasing authorities that allowed rapid and directed acquisition and avoided long contractual negotiations. In spite of this, there were evolving challenges as worldwide suppliers refused to ship materials without prepayment.

Government acquisition regulation requires government-purchasing agents to physically inspect delivered materials before authorizing the release of funds to pay for those materials. For those items being purchased from China and Asia, there are no US government-purchasing agents in China and Vietnam to inspect products and facilitate prepayment. This mandatory inspection requirement cannot be relegated to a third party acting on behalf of the US government. Therefore, we were now blocked from our primary source of consumable materials across the world. Our logistics team interviewed dozens of US manufacturers, and we were lectured repeatedly on the time and cost to establish US-based manufacturing capability. I was given a robust history lesson by multiple suppliers on the continued movement to "just in time" delivery and how it had affected the diminution of the American medical material manufacturing base.

It was at this point that it became clear to me that this type of material dependence on foreign manufacturers was a **fundamental national security risk**. Even if we could obtain contracts with foreign entities for materials, risk to those countries' own citizens made the completion of material delivery a sustained risk. I believed VHA would need to establish robust material stores in what we called readiness warehouses. This would require the support of the DOD's Defense Logistics Agency and would also require that we develop a model of material delivery from foreign sources that would bridge the possible implementation of the envisioned DPA authorities. It was hoped that the use of the DPA by the president would bring domestic production back to life.

A key to this effort to stabilize the supply chain was the secretary of the VA, Office of Strategic Partnerships under the direction and leadership of an extraordinarily talented leader by the name of Deborah Lafer Scher. Deborah is an extensively experienced coalition builder who has worked for two presidential administrations and four cabinet level secretaries. She was comfortable in high-stress environments and provided both the professionalism and possessed the worldwide contacts to stabilize a rapidly devolving situation. When she arrived to support the VHA in this effort, she already had over fifty corporate partners supporting various initiatives across VA.

Deborah had completed her undergraduate work in sociology and then received an MBA in finance from Columbia University Graduate School of Business. She had a long history of success in developing what are termed public-private and public-public partnerships that occur between government and private industry. Her skill would rapidly become invaluable to our sustained operations.

The VA office that Deborah led directly reports to the VA secretary and facilitates the myriad of relationships necessary to serve America's Veterans. Focus areas include public-private and public-public relationships with respect to potential donated buildings and ongoing research in emerging service-related threats to both service members and Veterans. As an aside, it is not unusual for a wealthy patriotic American citizen to donate financial or material items of value to the VHA in support of Veterans. The ability to complete those transactions and comply with complex law that protects the donating citizen, and the US government was Deborah's responsibility.

For a year prior to the pandemic, the Baylor, Scott & White Health system in Dallas attempted to donate a 1970's era unused hospital to the VHA. There was substantial concern on the part of the government because of the building's age. It was my opinion that the building would save the American taxpayer over five hundred million dollars in avoidance of the need to complete new construction in this community and would immediately deliver an inpatient Veteran care location in under-served north Dallas. The donated hospital would then allow VHA to expand the existing landlocked Dallas VAMC site once we had moved appropriate patients to the donated hospital location. As this donation progressed toward reality, there developed a profound sense of urgency to complete the donation in order to protect the Dallas VAMC from reaching overflow capacity of COVID-19 patients. The work of Deborah Scher's team to bring this donation to successful conclusion is a perfect example of the value of an office and a leader whose sole focus was to ensure these types of transactions were completed for the benefit of the American Veteran and the American taxpayer.

Deborah and I began regular phone consultations on the myriad of challenges that I faced as the pandemic progressed across the nation. It was great to have someone removed from VHA itself to discuss challenges and possible solutions with. She was always willing to work her rolodex of supportive partners to assist us if at all possible. We spent multiple calls each week reviewing the "pay in advance" problem for materials purchased overseas. Her team began working with VA legal counsel to examine options for this rapidly emerging challenge that threatened the stability of the entire VHA health care operation. She identified a potential relationship between the Governor of New Hampshire, Chris Sununu, and a well-known inventor and resident of New Hampshire, Dean Kamen.

Dean Kamen is a world-renowned engineer, inventor, and businessman who invented the personal transportation device known as the Segway and holds over one thousand patents, many of which are medically related, to include the first intravenous infusion pump as well as an insulin pump. Kamen has facilitated student learning in robotics using an organization that he developed. This organization is named "For Inspiration and Recognition of Science and Technology" (FIRST). This organization has sponsored thousands of American students' participation in robotics competition over the last twenty years.

Deborah discovered that Mr. Kamen had business relationships in China that could potentially be used to secure medical protective equipment and other health-related materials on a regular weekly delivery schedule to the state of New Hampshire. Deborah's office worked directly with the state of New Hampshire and with Dean Kamen's staff to leverage these relationships and bring much-needed supplies into the United States for VHA and America's Veterans. The system she developed would ensure these materials were paid for in advance and delivered to the state of New Hampshire on giant FedEx aircraft. The materials were personally paid for by this prolific American inventor. The entire cost of delivered materials was at Kamen's expense. The state of New Hampshire would then purchase the materials as they were unloaded and turned over to the state of New Hampshire, where US government inspectors then inspected and assured that the materials met federal safety and manufacturing guidelines. These materials could then transfer to VHA-contracted commercial transport vehicles and were moved across the nation to support ongoing VHA operations. Through Deborah's effective negotiation, all parties agreed to this convoluted arrangement. The first FedEx plane packed with 91,000 pounds of PPE arrived in New Hampshire on April 12, 2020.

It should be noted that Dean Kamen was at personal financial risk should any of these shipments fail to pass US government inspection. It should also be noted that Mr. Kamen is not in the consumable medical supply business. A year after this crisis, a media outlet criticized this arrangement and even questioned the patriotism of Mr. Kamen. I review the events here because there was real danger that the nation's largest health care system would run out of materials to protect the safety and wellbeing of vulnerable Veterans and hundreds of thousands of VHA employees, and Mr. Kamen, Governor Sununu, and all involved partners were essential in our ability to overcome this potential disaster and continue to operate.

This problem highlights what I believe is a monumental weakness in our nation's supply chain. This weakness is fixable in a number of ways. It is almost shameful that the nation's second-largest government agency and largest integrated health care system had to depend upon the patriotism, kindness, and generosity of a private US citizen who placed millions of his personal dollars at risk for months as the worldwide medical supply chain faltered. The effectiveness of this response was also dependent upon the support of a well-experienced state governor and his team of experts who understood the national risk in failure to supply these materials.

Some potential solutions are as follows:

First, the government could ensure that domestic-based manufacturing of these materials is constructed, developed, and sustained. This national security risk demands the development of a robust US manufacturing base for medical materials. If the nation cannot sustain this manufacturing base and is forced to purchase these materials around the world, then there must be a stockpiled and continuously sustained medical supply storage system that is robust enough to sustain itself many months or even years following a foreign supply chain disruption.

Fortunately, there is a model for just such a system within the Department of Defense. Following Operation Desert Storm in late 1990 and extending into February 1991, DOD faced similar supply chain challenges that included the absence of an industrial base agile enough to supply necessary materials to sustain the Persian Gulf War. After a thorough review by DOD and congressional hearings that reviewed in detail this problem, Congress passed the National Defense Authorization Act for 1992 and 1993 and identified multiple "war stopper" items that had been at risk during the short war that forced Iraq from its occupation of Kuwait.

The identified items were those that were in high demand during wartime but whose need reduced rapidly during peacetime. They included items, such as nerve agent antidote autoinjectors, chemical protective suits, gloves, and so on. The Defense Logistics Agency was authorized to purchase and manage these potential "war stopper" items with the support of American industry that would rotate and maintain the readiness of these supplies. The program also ensured the surge capacity of American industry that manufactured these items through sustained contracts. Over the years that this system has operated, additional materials have become part of this program to include some pharmaceuticals. It is an example of successful management of the supply chain that could be duplicated for the VA to obtain and manage medical materials previously discussed.

VHA purchases more than ten billion dollars annually of pharmaceuticals for Veterans, mostly through prime vendors (not directly from manufacturers). These pharmaceutical materials are delivered to VHA using a similar, just in time delivery process as described for other consumable supplies. Just as the consumable medical materials discussed previously, virtually all of the VHA's top one hundred-most used pharmaceutical agents are manufactured outside the United States.

As the pandemic accelerated, we recognized that large numbers of very seriously ill COVID-19 patients developed unstable diabetes mellitus during their most vulnerable stages of care. This exacerbation of newly developed diabetes was requiring large amounts of insulin usage in order to stabilize the patients' blood sugars. As the VHA consumed insulin in quantities never experienced before by the supply chain, for the first time, we recognized that virtually all insulin used in America is manufactured outside the United States. We also recognized that the rest of the world, including those nation's housing the manufacturers of insulin, were experiencing the same demand for medical materials and insulin as the US. We also began to recognize that even longtime American allies would protect their own citizens access to medication before allowing pharmaceutical shipments outside their borders. Those shipments would thus potentially deny lifesaving materials to their own citizens. As we recognized the lack of pharmaceutical manufacturing within the United States, we also realized that even the base chemicals or active pharmaceutical ingredients (APIs) that are combined into pharmaceutical agents were often unavailable in the United States. Data on this is difficult to find, but even the most optimistic reports suggest that less than 30 percent of API pharmaceutical materials are produced in the United States.[44]

The United States is the largest pharmaceutical market in the world, consuming about 500 billion dollars of pharmaceuticals each year. The world consumes about 1.2 trillion dollars of pharmaceuticals every year, so the US accounts for about 40 percent of the world's market. Five of the ten largest pharmaceutical companies in the world are headquartered in the United States, but manufacturing of their materials is not tracked transparently by the FDA. [45]

The American people remain vulnerable if supplies of medical material, pharmaceuticals, or even the base chemicals required for pharmaceutical manufacturing must be imported to the US from other nations, just like the 1991 recognition that supply chain stability is a potential war stopper.

If the VHA is to remain the nation's health care backstop, then the stockpiling and management of medical supply materials requires that the VHA abandon a just in time medical material delivery model and develop robust supply stockage that can sustain not only America's Veterans but also emergency supplies beyond the nation's strategic national stockpile and the DOD war stopper program. A robust and transparent dialogue must occur rapidly in order to ensure the safety of all Americans during the next once-in-a-hundred-year pandemic.

CHAPTER EIGHTEEN

Working at the Top of a Medical License In Order To Save Lives

VHA OPERATES AN "INTEGRATED" nationwide health care delivery system. As a Veteran who receives my healthcare at a VHA facility, I am assigned to a primary care delivery team that includes my provider and his support staff to include registered nurses. This is not dissimilar to what the civilian health care systems in the nation offers. What is different is the integration of social work, behavioral health providers, and clinical pharmacists into the primary care team. This team-based approach allows the VHA to deliver full care integration for all of my health care needs as a Veteran. An example of this care integration is as follows.

Let's say a Veteran receiving care outside the VHA with prostate cancer, asthma, and type two (adult onset) diabetes is having trouble getting his cancer specialist, pulmonary specialist, and internist to coordinate their individual care of his complex pharmacology needs. This has caused multiple phone calls from the Veteran to his providers in an effort to control his diabetes while the pulmonary specialist titrates his asthma control meds that cause a rise in his blood sugar. There is no forum for his other providers to even be aware of this challenge without the patient initiating contact with each one individually. Calls are made by the Veteran to each provider; support staff record a message and promise a call back with the provider's nurse. The nurse calls in forty-eight hours and then again records the problem and states the provider will be informed. The nurse then promises a call back within forty-eight hours. Four to five days has now elapsed, resulting in progressive worsening of the patient's diabetes.

Now let's compare that to how the VHA handles it: In the fully integrated system, the primary care team clinical pharmacist is informed immediately when potential conflicting pharmaceutical problems like this are occurring, usually before the medication is even prescribed. The clinical pharmacist arranges for a weekly proactive teleconference with this Veteran, during which the patient and pharmacist reviews the Veteran's diabetes control (using home-based testing), and they work to deconflict the medications. The pharmacist then informs all providers using group messaging of identified challenges and recommended medication changes. The pharmacist then confirms by telephone, email, or text to the Veteran that his care team is aligned on all decisions that have been made. We call this model of care, allowing the provider, in this case, the clinical pharmacist, to work at the "top of their license" and truly take on the leadership role they were trained for but rarely asked to do outside the VHA. This model of care is facilitated by the integration of the care team but also enabled by the "federal supremacy" of the VHA, which allows individually licensed state providers to work across state lines regardless of their location. Let me explain this further:

In the United States, all professional medical practitioners, even at VHA, are licensed by their state medical boards. There are substantial nuances to each state's scope of services that a pharmacist, RN, MD/DO, PA, psychologist, or social worker, and so on can provide in their state, but those nuances are erased to a common scope of practice within the federal VHA delivery system. This system (enabled by federal law) allows a provider in New York to manage a patient (similar to what I have described) who may reside in New York but spend time in Arizona for part of the year. This is often accomplished by telemedicine. This allows the patient to sustain the benefit of their regular care team that knows the complexity of their care needs well. It also prevents the need for the Veteran to find a new care team while in Arizona, fragmenting his or her care. This ability to practice across state lines occurs for patients enrolled in VHA care regardless of the patient or provider's location.

Most Americans are highly mobile, and as we age, many Americans who live in northern climates and who are able, travel to and reside in warmer climates during the winter months. The pandemic facilitated the expansion of remote work and prompted substantial relocation of many Americans, fracturing medical care continuity for many of those who relocated. There has been much written about telemedicine during the pandemic; bringing care to the patient and not needing to bring the patient to brick and mortar facilities is convenient for patients and promotes more effective, uninterrupted, and seamless contact between provider teams and the patient. The unfortunate nature of individual state medical licensure creates significant barriers to this potential continuity of care when and where a patient needs help.

All Americans deserve the benefit of care regardless of their location in proximity to their provider. One of the significant lessons learned of this pandemic is that moving to reciprocity of state licensure across all state lines has the potential to unify care delivery and create a more seamless system. By this, I am suggesting that if my provider has an established relationship with me, she should be able to continue my care regardless of what state I am temporarily or even permanently located in, including the ability to order pharmaceuticals and diagnostic testing when appropriate. The alternative to this model would be a federal rather than a state licensure for professional health practitioners. This is currently the model for the prescription of controlled substances, where each provider must have a federal controlled substance license (Drug Enforcement Administration license). There is substantial value however, to a system of state oversight of provider quality, competency, and discipline when necessary. All of these could be retained at the state level with the suggested reciprocity concept and would expand the ability to provide continuity of care to all Americans beyond what Veterans enrolled in the VHA or DOD delivery system currently experience. A secondary value of this proposed system would be to avoid surging demand of temporary residents on an existing community health system during certain times of the year. Finally, this proposed reciprocity would place substantial pressure on the telemedicine industry to accelerate advances in technology that enable this care model.

It is important to recognize that VHA is a unique provider of care when compared to other American health care systems. VHA inherits as a service member leaves uniformed service a lifelong provider relationship with its Veteran patients. That lifelong relationship creates unique responsibilities unlike traditional insurance plans that move providers and patients into and out of participating relationships. Those movements have the potential to fragment patient care relationships. The ability

WORKING AT THE TOP OF A MEDICAL LICENSE IN ORDER TO SAVE LIVES

to integrate care and the ability to leverage long-term provider-patient relationships should be recognized in the improved complex care outcomes VHA has demonstrated.

This "working to the top of a professional's license" concept arose immediately during the early days of the pandemic as the VHA began to recognize the complexity of ventilator management on intubated and ventilator-dependent patients across the VHA. When a patient can no longer breathe without mechanical support, a tube is inserted through their mouth into their trachea. A machine is hooked to the tube, and the ventilator then provides positive pressure to force oxygen into and waste gases out of the patient's lungs. Prior to the pandemic, the insertion of the tube (intubation) and the setup of the breathing machine was usually done by an anesthesiologist or certified registered nurse anesthetist (CRNA) who were called to the patient's bedside. A CRNA is an advanced practice registered nurse (APRN) trained with special expertise in the delivery of anesthesia services. These providers usually hold advanced degrees in this specialty.

This process, although very intense, usually happens quite quickly. In the case of COVID-19 patients, however, we found that ventilator stabilization of a patient could take an extraordinary amount of time and was unlike most patient conditions our providers had experienced, including patients remaining unpredictably stable even with very low levels of oxygen in their blood. This meant that intubations started taking longer, and we needed more of them more frequently, straining our limited supply of anesthesia providers.

As we reviewed this, we found tremendous variation across the VHA in how CRNAs and physician anesthesiologists were working together within their scope of practice. This included variation based on state authorities as well as variation even in individual medical center's scope of practice (sometimes even changing based on time of day), thus reducing the continuity and efficiency of care across the system. We could find no difference in the quality of care or outcome of patients when we reviewed the safety of care based on whether this work was delivered to the patient by the CRNA or physician anesthesiologist.

Multiple states across the nation recognized these same challenges and the rapidly expanding need for airway management expertise at the bedside, and in recognition of this challenge, I issued an emergency but temporary declaration of "full independent practice authority" to nurse anesthetists (CRNAs). This caused substantial external and internal dialogue by organizations representing each profession, a dialogue that continues to occur even these many months later. The VHA must formalize and make permanent that decision of full practice authority for CRNAs as the pandemic comes to a conclusion. There is substantial value to aligning this decision to a previous decision that created independent full practice authority to other advance practice nurses in the VHA in 2016. In 2016, CRNAs were specifically excluded because the case for full practice authority for anesthesia providers had not been made effectively. The pandemic has now identified the need for this full practice authority in order to deliver effective and timely care to sick patients and proven CRNAs' capability to do so.

It is notable that full independent practice authority for the CRNA is an Army, Navy, and Air Force medicine standard. Most combat anesthesia has been provided by CRNAs since the beginning of the war on terrorism. An Army Forward Surgical Team is staffed only with CRNAs, and care for the critically wounded in those combat care units has delivered unprecedented combat wounded survival. Surely, these providers can continue to offer the same care to our nation's Veterans.

The added value of engaging all our anesthesia providers across the VHA system to the full value of their licensure was the ability to safely repurpose anesthesia machines used in the operating rooms as dual-use ICU ventilators. These machines are highly sophisticated and capable of acting as a ventilator while also delivering anesthesia-inhaled gasses during surgery. This repurposing to bedside, non-anesthesia care could only have occurred with the cooperative and combined intellect of the VHA MD/DO anesthesiologists and CRNAs' support of bedside respiratory therapists. As my decision for full independent practice authority was being debated inside and outside the VHA, at the bedside, the VHA care teams continued to work seamlessly. This is a testament to their professionalism and commitment to their Veteran and civilian patients.

I have previously discussed the movement of nursing and support personnel from ambulatory care to support the provision of inpatient critical care. I have also discussed that this required significant retraining and refreshing of skills. The ability to meet ongoing demand for continued ambulatory care from Veterans was a prime concern as these employees were repositioned. VHA's model as an integrated health care system was able to support the ongoing health needs of our patients even when the pandemic interrupted the ability to deliver that care face to face. We were most concerned that the reduction of in-person care and the safety concerns expressed by patients and families who were unwilling to continue care in a face-to-face manner due to a fear of infection would result in a delayed response of our providers to new onset patient symptoms, diseases, and even the delayed diagnosis of cancers or failure to recognize the recurrence of cancers. As an example, the VHA has very high levels of cancer screening for women Veterans for breast and cervical cancer, and the concerns were based upon the possibility that changes in ambulatory care availability would reduce screening and inevitably lead to delayed diagnosis of potential carcinomas. This potential tidal wave of delayed, deferred, and undiagnosed care remains a significant and newly recognized risk of the pandemic across the nation. Increased patient visits to the ER for poorly managed cardiovascular conditions has resulted in a rapid expansion across VHA of telemedicine and even digitally enabled home-based patient monitoring for these conditions. However, we still have a long road to deliver the robust capabilities possible under a health system transformation as complex as telemedicine could become.

VHA had been a national leader in telemedicine care delivery for more than a decade prior to the onset of the pandemic. This has included development of a nationwide tele-ICU care delivery service to deliver critical care professional expertise to remote areas where medical and surgical intensivists are not readily available on site. This work is enabled by technology that enables an intensivist anywhere in the VHA system to interact with a patient and care staff hundreds of miles away at the patient's bedside. This model of care has also been adopted in partnership with the Air Force. The application of this technology-enabled care allows VHA to partner with the Air Force to deliver ICU care in facilities where the Air Force is unable to provide on-site critical care expertise 24/7.

Prior to the pandemic, most patients desired face-to-face appointments with their providers. The growth of "technology-enabled" remote patient visits grew incrementally prior to the pandemic until safety concerns regarding face-to-face visits arose during the pandemic. As these concerns grew, telemedicine visits as an effective option for ambulatory care grew exponentially. Behavioral health providers were leaders in the adoption of this technology, and the ability of psychologists, psychiatrists, and psychiatric social workers to interact with patients using video and audio conferencing in real-time from a patient's home had significant and previously unrecognized value. This included visibility into the patient's family dynamics and living situation amongst others and also allowed even physically remote family members to join a telemedicine visit (with the patient's permission). The provision of these services was accepted by both providers and patients with high levels of satisfaction in both groups.

This explosive growth in these technology services taxed the VA Office of Information Technology to field and support large numbers of providers working from home. It protected the provider workforce but created a dynamic situation to provide a cyber protected IT environment that ensured the patient's digital records were secure. As the pandemic began, Jim Gfrerer asked during a regularly scheduled meeting between him and me what volume of providers would need to be accommodated remotely on the secure system simultaneously. I gave an estimate of the volume, and one year later, OIT was servicing ten times my estimate with sometimes tens of thousands of simultaneous users providing care using technology-enabled visits.

The second piece of this remote delivery system was the ability of Veterans to utilize this system from their own devices, especially iPads. These highly mobile and easy-to-use devices were purchased by VHA in bulk from Apple, and more than 100,000 were distributed to at-risk and even homeless Veterans to ensure their continued connectivity to VHA providers. Deborah Sher supported this effort by partnering with all major cellular providers to provide cellular-enabled services even in areas where internet was not available. This cooperative alliance with Apple, T-Mobile, Verizon, AT&T, and Sprint was unique and reflected these companies' commitment to supplying seamless care to Americas' Veterans. T-Mobile should especially be recognized for their extraordinary leadership in this area. Their willingness to provide tools that allowed Veterans to communicate with VHA providers while not consuming data volume in their monthly plans was unique and a model for other cellular providers. This reflected what Deborah Sher often said: "There are people who want to help; you just have to ask."

One final note: Understanding Veteran satisfaction with these changes was essential to defining the future of care using digitally-enabled visits conducted remotely. We found through nearly continuous measurement that Veterans were highly satisfied with visits that allowed video transmission so that there was the ability to see and react to human facial expressions and body language from both the provider and patient. Telephonic (audio only) visits were accepted well for less intense or less emotionally stressful interactions such as prescription refills. During the months when COVID-19 rates dropped, telephonic visits dropped rapidly as well. Video visits, conducted in real-time, remained stable and grew in the number of completed visits regardless of COVID-19 volume as they reflected the value of multisensory human interaction.

These lessons on the value of video-based and enabled visits would expand even into the application of this technology to the bedside of patients who were precluded from family visits or even as they experienced end-of-life care. The ability to restore, in some measure, the extraordinary value of having a family member at the bedside, even remotely, supported the emotional well-being of patients, their families, and their care delivery team.

CHAPTER NINETEEN

Dying Alone, Grieving, and the Idea of Stability in Life

DYING ALONE . . . I've learned a myriad of lessons about life in caring for patients over my decades of delivering patient care. One of the most important is the value of family and loved ones to support a patient through the most difficult of health challenges, including the approach of death (as I discussed at the end of the last chapter). As VHA considered the need to protect vulnerable Veterans and our staff from COVID-19, I made the decision to temporarily stop all visitors entering our facilities. End-of-life visitation was allowed on a case-by-case basis, but most families expressed concern about being exposed to the virus by their family member and the need to quarantine (based on CDC guidance) for ten to fourteen days after exposure. This resulted in the loss of family as important members of individual patient's care teams. Family members of critically ill patients bring context and history to the care team when at the bedside. They help bring the patient's life into context and can often speak for the patient. It is not unusual for busy critical care teams to view patients they have never met before the current hospitalization as clinically complex disease processes rather than as a mother, father, sister, brother, aunt, uncle, and so on.

A spouse at the bedside grieves impending loss and relates to bedside caregivers the nuances of a relationship and lifetime of companionship that helps the care team process and humanizes the impending loss of a loved one.

While in Afghanistan in 2003 and 2004, I was blessed with an exceedingly experienced trauma care team at all levels from surgeon, internist, nurse, medic, respiratory therapist, and so on. At the bedside were decades of experienced professionals caring for major trauma. As we experienced major battles and significant US casualties, I began to witness the emotional trauma of the injuries and deaths upon the care delivery team. We opened an intimate dialogue with each other about this unique emotional connection to our patients. One highly experienced trauma surgeon related the emotional pain he was experiencing and said, "In my civilian coverage of ERs and trauma delivery systems, I could always find a way to emotionally separate myself from the victim, even young victims. They were drunk, they initiated a fight, or they should have never been in the area where they were shot. Sometimes it wasn't fair in the way I viewed the victim, but it allowed me to work with major injury and death and remain objective. Here, in Afghanistan, every one of these victims is my brother or sister. I can't separate myself from them; I am connected emotionally to every one of them." And with that, he began to weep. I listened quietly and realized that our brotherhood of service would connect us forever, even to those we could not save.

On a difficult night in Afghanistan with multiple US casualties in the ER, the Army medical care team recognized that one of the service members we had received was slipping toward death from multiple gunshot wounds. Two of his unit members had remained at the bedside, and before I realized what was happening, one of them dialed the soldier's wife in the United States on a satellite phone. He explained the gravity of the situation to her and asked that she just speak to her husband as he then placed the phone gently against her husband's ear. He cautioned that her husband wouldn't be able to verbally respond. As he slipped further toward death, she was there the entire time, speaking to him through her own tears and profound unimaginable emotion. We all were humbled and brought to tears by the love and compassion she expressed in her words to her husband. As death overtook her husband, the soldier holding the phone removed it from her spouse's ear and handed it immediately to me to relate his passing. There are no words to convey the sense of loss our entire team experienced that night. Her telephonic presence and grace in thanking us for our effort to save him was a testament to the strength of the American military spouse. The warmth of her presence helped each of us process the loss of an extraordinary American hero.

As we made the decision to remove family from the bedside of VHA patients in the early stages of the pandemic, even for those critically ill, I reflected on that night in Afghanistan and the spouse who delivered such grace and strength through a satellite phone and the profound implications of what we were doing in order to protect family members and VHA staff. I also recognized the toll these decisions would have on the families of Veteran patients and our caregivers.

One of the primary reasons given by employees when they join the VHA is the chance to care for America's heroes and their families. About one-third of VHA employees are Veterans themselves. These extraordinary employees most often describe their continued government service as continuing the mission they had performed in uniform. Those non-Veteran VHA employees relate to the Veteran patient and family because their spouse, dad, mom, brother, or sister served in uniform, and they just want to serve them. To say this VHA care team is a unique family, tied by a sense of service, is completely accurate. To say that the sense of brotherhood reflected that night in the Afghanistan ER persists at the bedside of patients in the VHA is also accurate.

Following the decision that precluded family visits to the bedside of COVID-19 patients, we began to hear stories of VHA staff sitting at the bedside of critically ill patients, holding a patient's hand, and providing the presence of another compassionate human being. Often the person who volunteered to sit at the bedside was an ambulatory care nurse who had been retrained and repurposed to become part of the critical care team. This not only freed the critical care team to perform other tasks but preserved the humanity and connection between the care team and their patients.

Over my time in combat, I have had patients die while I listened to their last words and struggle with their last breaths. These are sacred times and a privilege and deep honor to be present in those final moments. As we experienced those same moments in the pandemic, we realized that bringing family to the bedside, even using digitalized technology, was absolutely necessary. We were able to provide iPads to the COVID-19 nursing units and encouraged families to interact with their hospitalized Veteran using these devices. As death approached for some of these patients, we facilitated the family being present virtually through these technologies with a staff member interpreting what was occurring in the care of their loved one. These were indescribably difficult moments for both the family and for the care delivery team.

There is no doubt that the physical presence of a loving family member would have been better. We had made this decision to bar visitation in order to protect family members and protect and preserve our staff as we worked to limit the potential spread of the virus. Some, looking through the lens of hindsight, will criticize this decision, but fear of contracting COVID-19 had already reduced hospital visitation in most other situations. I discussed the decision to limit visitation with the leadership of the Veterans Benefit Administration and the VA's National Cemetery Administration (NCA). The director of the NCA pointed out that one-third of funerals for Veterans at federal cemeteries were being conducted as direct internments (immediate burials) because families stated they had no one that would be attending the funeral. This occurred because of fear of transmission of the virus. There was not fear of viral transmission from the deceased but from other mourners. As we consider the events of 2020 and 2021, the loneliness of COVID-19-induced death, and the inability to grieve and express a profound sense of loss of a loved one are lasting emotional injuries that will take years for each of us who have lived these events to reconcile.

Over my military career, I have lost soldiers under my command to disease, combat, accident, and suicide. In early 2003, as I mobilized a US Army Reserve combat hospital at Ft McCoy Wisconsin, we prepared soldiers for combat deployment by administering a large number of vaccinations, including anthrax and smallpox. One of the 548 soldiers I had mobilized from the Army Reserve had an unrecognized immune deficit, and in response to these vaccinations, this twenty-two-year-old soldier died within a few days of vaccination. In every one of these cases of loss, including this twenty-two-year-old soldier, we were able to pause to grieve the loss. We stopped whatever we were doing, including preparation for wartime deployment, for a brief period to reflect on the loss of our valued friend, brother, or sister in arms and grieve.

In wartime, all combat losses eventually come through the medical care system. Even combat losses were followed by a period of grieving. Following the death of a seriously wounded service member, what followed was incredibly powerful and reflected Americans' most cherished values and traditions.

The movement of the deceased service members' remains were powerfully emotional events where a lost service member who had been placed in a transport coffin was draped in an American flag. The service member was then transported by military ambulance from the hospital to a waiting C-17 aircraft for the flight to repatriate the service member with their country and reunite with their family. As this movement of the deceased service member took place, the route of the ambulance from the hospital to the aircraft, was lined on a completely impromptu basis by soldiers, sailors, marines, and airmen who stood shoulder to shoulder along the route, saluting the lost brother or sister in arms as the vehicle moved slowly toward the flight line.

Most of those lining the roadway would then fall in and walk behind the ambulance to the aircraft and perform a final salute as the flag-draped coffin was moved into the aircraft. This grieving was often accompanied by the playing of "Amazing Grace" on bagpipes by a service member who would walk directly behind the ambulance. There was grief, healing, and respect for life. There was also respect expressed for service to the nation during these periods of mostly impromptu formalized grieving. These events had value to those of us who

SAVE EVERY LIFE YOU CAN

remained behind and allowed for some modicum of closure and healing.

As the pandemic progressed in March 2020, the VHA experienced the death of its first employee due to COVID-19. As the pandemic was spreading rapidly, for the first time in my career, there was no ability to pause the organization in order to grieve the loss of that employee. We could not travel, and the quarantine of fellow employees prevented group reflection of the tragic loss. The sheer operational pace prevented the expression of our emotions. I asked for a picture of the employee and placed that picture under the glass top of the large conference table in my office. Soon, the entire conference table would be covered in pictures. The VHA would experience the death of more than 145 employees to COVID-19 over the next fifteen months. For most of those lost, we did not know if they had been infected at work or outside work from family members or acquaintances. Operationally, this distinction was important because we wanted to ensure we were providing as much protection to employees as possible in the workplace, but in the end, each loss was felt the same.

Some will believe we did not protect workers well enough, and I am respectful of those who believe that. But the point I am trying to make here is that we could not grieve. And I believe grieving facilitates the ability to move forward. It also supports and sustains our individual resilience.

During a particularly brutal day in Afghanistan in 2004, we lost six American soldiers in a single horrific event. The leadership of the Combined Joint Task Force was devastated by these losses, and the sadness was palpable as the leadership team met with then Brigadier General (one star) Lloyd Austin, our commander. The leadership team was assembled in a conference room he used for meeting with the senior leaders. The temperature was always cool in the mud-walled room. Lloyd Austin is a tall and imposing figure, and I will never forget his words that day, spoken slowly in his characteristic deep and commanding voice. I am sure that I paraphrase these words from nearly twenty years ago.

"There are events in combat that just make you feel like you are frozen in place. But our mission demands that you must move forward. The nation expects that. And I expect that of you. We cannot stop, no matter how much it feels right to do so. Sometimes it takes the physical act of digging your heels in the sand and just leaning forward. Today is one of those days. So, dig your heels in, and let's continue to move."

As we experienced the loss of the first VHA employee and then another, and then another, I realized we could not pause in order to appropriately grieve those losses. I asked for the VA chief of chaplains, Juliana Lesher, to join us at our daily nationwide operational updates conducted from the operations center. I also asked her to address the entire team on our mounting losses each week with a weekly reflection. I believed it was Chaplain Lesher who could help this team dig in their heels and lean forward to continue the mission.

Chaplain Lesher was serving at that time as the national director of VA chaplain's services, leading a staff of more than 800 chaplains assigned to individual medical centers. With a PhD in organizational leadership and a master's degree in divinity, her calm and direct communication style was perfect for this mission.

I have always believed that there are certain "anchors" that stabilize and protect each of us as the ill wind of life's challenges are blown toward us. Those anchors, among others, include the presence of our significant partner or spouse, family, community, source of income, sense of productive work, health, and spiritual and organizational faith. I define each of these very broadly, and for service members, their family members may include the members of their assigned military units. We also know that spiritual faith is an incredibly deep and often unshakable anchor that service members resort to when facing life-threatening situations. But faith may also refer to faith in my employer (organizational) to do the right thing for me or my family when I am meeting a personal life challenge. Each of these things anchor us. For those with multiple anchors, they can generally demonstrate the resiliency we admire when a significant challenge is confronted. For those without these anchors, even the most insignificant life challenge can be overwhelming.

I have been impressed with the ability of those with deep spiritual faith to sustain themselves while facing the breakup of a marriage or even the death of a spouse, family member, or child. Their ability to express grief and place the event they face in some context that sustains them is to be admired. I remain concerned that for those without anchors, there is an inability to maintain their footing when even experiencing a minor setback in their lives. I ask you to consider those individuals in your own lives who become overwhelmed and struggle to function when what most would consider a minor life event occurs. In my experience, those individuals usually are struggling with a lack of life's "anchors."

Chaplain Lesher and I began to meet weekly and discuss her impression of the morale and resilience of the VHA workforce and my senior leadership team. I was impressed with her knowledge and connection to the VHA chaplains assigned and located at each VHA medical center. Those chaplains' role in an individual hospital is to support the spiritual needs of patients, families, and caregivers as they faced life's difficult challenges and crises. They also provide support to the professional staff at the medical center. These are trained providers of non-denominational faith who arrive in those situations when most of us are at a loss for words. They are often meeting those in need of support for the first time. In the VHA, they are connected by the bond of service I referenced in previous pages. Juliana related story after story of the resilience of our workforce coming from the medical center staff chaplains. She expressed concern for the ability of the workforce to sustain for the long term but was steadfast in her confidence in the ability of the VHA workforce to perform their ongoing duties with excellence.

Throughout the pandemic, I sought input from every senior leader about the resilience of the workforce and tried to discuss with each of them their ability to sustain their own effort needed to keep moving forward. Of all their input, I found that from Juliana, it was extraordinarily helpful as I contemplated what actions I needed to take to effectively support the workforce.

CHAPTER TWENTY

Mitigating Isolation of the Workforce

As the pandemic accelerated, there was significant concern by employees at all levels about exposure to this deadly virus. Our first mission is to care for sick, ill, or injured Veterans. That mission requires that we serve most often in direct contact with our very ill patients and that we are available on demand for emergent health problems irrespective of the risk. In early March 2020, we began considering the ability of the VA information technology systems to effectively accommodate large numbers of remote workers who might be able to perform their work from home. This began with concerns about the Veteran Crisis Line operations, which are housed in facilities that congregate those employees who answer thousands of calls from potentially suicidal Veterans each day in three unique locations around the country. These employees sit side by side in small cubicles; therefore, our concern was a widespread infection of these essential employees. Should this workforce develop high numbers of COVID-19, the resultant quarantine would decimate the ability to deliver timely crisis telephone support.

Our building engineers had examined the facilities where these three call centers operate, and there were few options to increase the safety of this vital workforce. By the middle of

March 2020, I was convinced that moving this workforce to a remote model of work from home was essential to protect both them and the integrity of the crisis line operation. My concern was the adequacy of the information technology platforms to accept thousands of employees working from home. We could not afford to collapse or degrade this system, or we would expose the potential high risk of suicide patients to inaccessible support.

About this time, a nontraditional media source began a short series of reports echoing concerns of non-clinical and even some clinical employees of VHA expressing anonymous concerns about their safety and inability to receive approval for work from home. The VA Office of Information Technology, concurrently with these media reports, had stabilized the expansion of our "work from home" IT platforms, and by the third week of March, I was able to release directives approving the broad implementation of telework for those employees not essential to actual bedside care. This nontraditional media source and a regional media outlet suggested in their March 25, 2020, report that it was their reporting that had forced my decision. In fact, the decision reflected the VA ability to assure safety of Veterans and our ability to perform our mission while at the same time protecting our employees as much as was possible. I relate this level of detail only to reflect the constant tension with media reporting that, however intentioned, added to the stress on our workforce and had the potential to profoundly reduce employees' trust in senior leadership. This level of scrutiny of management decisions is rarely directed to health systems outside government. Even within government, VA is often singled out for significant scrutiny of many, if not most, decisions. The ability of leaders to make informed decisions is often impacted by this constant media noise. This level of review, in this instance, is the author's perception that this type of reporting reduces employee confidence in leadership.

This decision for telework directed to the operating units in the field caused additional decisions on telework for our central office employees whose jobs were administrative and were never in contact with actual patients. The most senior VHA leadership team decided that because of the unique nature of the challenges we were facing and the pervasive culture of group problem-solving across our team that we would continue to perform face-to-face work while instituting robust efforts to limit large congregations of the team where physical distancing was not possible. About twenty senior leaders of VHA central office continued to come to work every day over the next eighteen months. None of us became infected with COVID-19 throughout this entire period in spite of a significant percentage whose families had become infected. This causes some consideration on the value of dispersing the workforce and if it really actually protected the workforce. In spite of that commentary, more than one hundred thousand VHA employees from central office and the field operating units began work from home across the entire system. For the vast majority, their productivity remained very high, and the quality of their work remained excellent. For those of us still in central office, a building designed for thousands of government employees that had been in use for over one hundred years, the hallways became eerily silent and dark, traversed only by the few who remained in person.

These decisions created a unique challenge for a team of leaders accustomed to walking around and interacting with employees at their workstations. We developed, in response to this dispersal of employees, "town hall" live video broadcasts for the dispersed workforce and accepted questions from remote employees. We increased the frequency of my two-minute videos and worked to answer every email sent to me with concerns, anticipating wide dissemination of the responses. Jon Jensen began his in-depth "Chats with the Chief" broadcasts to keep the workforce connected and engaged and provided a weekly email message to all VHA employees. During all of this, Jim Gfrerer's OIT team kept access to the secure information and communication system stable and accessible. This unique and productive partnership between IT leadership and the VHA remains essential to the VHA's continued success.

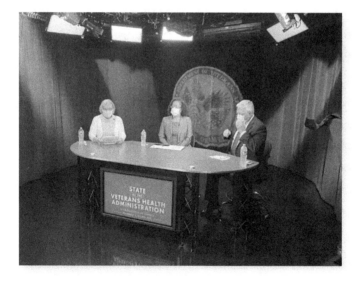

P7: VHA employee townhall broadcast. Pictured are the author, Renee Oshinski, chief of operations, and Kam Matthews, chief medical officer.

There were, during this time, leaders who were concerned that their voices were not heard. We were in the midst of a cultural transformation toward high reliability and implementing a zero-patient harm health care environment. This was in an effort to reduce medical care process errors and improve reliability in patient outcomes, the end result being an enhancement of Veteran trust in VHA. This transformation is dependent upon the training and coaching of leaders and personnel to recognize that creating an environment that identifies the role of each member of the team in safe and high-quality patient outcomes is each of their primary responsibility. That training and coaching had always been conducted in person and often even conducted in one-on-one training. Never had it been conducted virtually.

One of the great challenges of the inability to get trainers into a hospital was a slowdown in the implementation of this essential cultural change. Sustaining the trust of the American Veteran and the American people was dependent on this level of reliability. The High Reliability transformation training and implementation team, under the leadership of retired Navy Captain Gerry Cox, MD and William Patterson, MD, network director at VISN 15, had worked to create effective remote learning modules that supported the ongoing effort and maintained momentum in this work. These were valiant and innovative efforts, but there was no substitute for shoulder-to-shoulder training and mentoring. Gerry and Bill were excellent about ensuring I heard their team's voice and their concerns in this effort. I remain convinced that the restoration of the VHA's ability to earn and sustain the trust of the American Veteran directly related to the reliability and safe outcome of all our processes. The work of this team remains the bedrock of that effort and a model for all American health care systems.

As the pandemic wore on, it became apparent to me that my continued leadership effectiveness required resumption of travel to medical centers significantly challenged and in the midst of the COVID-19 response. To reduce risk, we attempted to create a travel model where we limited those traveling with me as much as possible. We developed protocols of rapid COVID-19 testing as we arrived at each site to ensure we were not transmitting COVID-19 to the medical center leadership, patients, or employees. In addition, we were each tested every week as we returned from travel by the chief medical officer of the Washington, DC, VA medical center. Using this model, we pledged to continue travel and demonstrate our support for those employees deep in the fight against the virus. Through these efforts, we also attempted to ensure that we did not consume resources necessary for patient care or employee protection.

My first pandemic-related trip was in May 2020 to two Chicago area VAMCs to review the performance of a newly deployed mobile intensive care unit that we had purchased during the pandemic and assess firsthand the impact of the pandemic on the workforce. For a leader accustomed to hundreds of travel engagements each year, the inability to travel during the first months of 2020 was a challenge to continued connection to the workforce and my basic principle of leaders being on the front line of employee challenges. This was a lesson learned from the earliest stages of my work career (the reader should review the lessons learned from the Safety Patrol story in chapter two).

Chicago was chosen because the ability to provide expanding amounts of critical care services was being tested at this site. The operating model we were developing allowed this new mobile unit to remain with the manufacturer who was responsible to sustain all the operating systems until we needed the capability. The twenty-ICU bed facility was then transported by the manufacturer to the location where it was needed. The manufacturer was also responsible to establish and bring the unit to operational readiness within a matter of days. The reader should return to my review of the problems recognized in the conversion of major city conference centers into acute care hospitals and their inability to deliver critical care services and sustain patient care continuity. It was the VHA plan to collocate these new mobile facilities on the property of a VA medical center and utilize the hospital staffing and logistics system to sustain operations.

We learned several lessons from the first actual patient use of this mobile capability in Chicago. These included the process of transporting critically ill patients outside, even across a parking lot, is very difficult and fraught with safety challenges. We, therefore, concluded that the mobile facility should be located as close to the medical center ER as possible. Even a few hundred feet made a difference. This mobile facility generated its own oxygen and purified its own water. The technology included in these mobile units was so advanced and robust that we could deliver water clean enough for even dialysate (highly purified water) for patients who needed kidney dialysis, a not uncommon occurrence in critically ill patients.

This mobile technology has now been expanded in the VHA to ensure there is the ability to deploy at least one of these units in each of the four regions of the country simultaneously. What was more difficult than we expected was to provide trained critical care staffing already competency-validated on the complex equipment in these mobile units. The VHA is actively engaged in the process of developing a rotational critical care emergency response workforce that ensures that a medical center requesting one of these units is not additionally tasked to staff or train on the functions of the mobile unit upon arrival. A medical center already overwhelmed needs help in all areas, not additional tasks to complete.

As I completed each of these visits around the country, there was a uniform and consistent message every bedside care employee that I met gave. First, they were not taking time off for earned vacation because their team and their Veteran patients needed them. Second, for those who had been infected with COVID-19, they had each pleaded with their managers to come back to work early because they absolutely believed their teams caring for infected patients needed them. Third, the loneliness of working completely gowned, masked, and gloved on a prolonged and sustained basis for months was personally difficult for each of them. The inability to express emotions from behind their PPE was weighing on every one of them. Many of them who were new hires to the VHA identified the extraordinary expertise of senior VHA nurses as a huge and valuable resource to their individual development as competent bedside providers.

For those employees who were more senior in their careers, I asked how long they could keep going. All of them, in every visit, said they would think about that when this pandemic was over, but for now, they were completely focused on saving every life they could. Over the calendar years 2020 and 2021, retirements at the VHA reached record low numbers among all categories of employees, from nurses to housekeepers. This team and mission-focused allegiance was unique in my nonuniformed career experience and mimicked the comradery and cohesiveness of combat-deployed military units.

It was also extraordinary the number of patient-engaged employees who stated during these visits their profound motivation to our mission to "save every life I can," a statement similar to what I had stated months before during a HOC meeting with senior leaders conducted very early in the pandemic response, and the title of this book. In my leadership career, I have rarely been so connected to a leadership philosophy that so adeptly characterized the response of this entire agency. From the frontline screener at a hospital to the secretary of the agency, every action was oriented to maximize the preservation of life.

We continued the recording of daily videos on each of these trips. They were always impromptu and recorded on handheld cell phones. Each stressed what we were seeing during the visit and the messages we were hearing from the employees we were in contact with. I underline here that if you are a leader, you do not need a media team to reach your employees—one person with a cell phone is what we used.

We recorded one of these videos from the "interstitial space" between the floors of the New Orleans VHA hospital. Interstitial space is literally a miniature floor inserted between two floors of a building. It can be a crawl space in height or even six feet of vertical space. These spaces are expensive to build but allow the placement of plumbing, electricity, heating, cooling, and cabling for data transmission to occur in easily accessible space. The transformation of a care delivery room above or below this space can occur without disrupting patient care being delivered in a patient's treatment room. The VHA has had an ongoing and, at times, animated discussion about the value of this space for decades. During the pandemic, those buildings where interstitial space existed between floors could be transformed with negative airflow technology almost overnight. For those buildings without this space, windows or walls needed to have holes placed in them to create negative airflow in order to improve patient and staff safety. It was important to our facility engineers that I fully comprehended the value of this space in our buildings. I can honestly report that I spent more time in building interstitial space than any previous VHA leader. So, in recognition of those visits, I recorded a video from one of these spaces so that every employee had the chance to understand the complexity of the changes we were undertaking (and lessons learned) in order to deliver a safe environment of care.

Other videos highlighted the local team's commitment and unique stories about heroic acts that had occurred at the location where we were visiting. Universally, when these videos aired across the entire system, I received hundreds of emails asking for our next trip to be to whatever hospital the email sender was employed at. They always invited me to their hospital to see what great work they and their team were doing. Pride in service was everywhere throughout the system. Pride in quality of care was palpable in every team member.

During many of these visits to medical centers, the topic of employee death was often raised, sometimes by me during conversations with groups of employees. In every one of these discussions, there was an acknowledgment by the bedside care employees that health care delivery was sometimes very dangerous work, especially during a pandemic. There was also a myriad of personal stories about each of those who were lost and always a reflection on the loss their families were experiencing. I didn't need to say much in response to these emotion and tear-filled discussions except how honored I was to know the lost employee through their words.

I am convinced that the extraordinarily bitter politicization of the pandemic public health and rapidly evolving patient care processes that extended from mask-wearing to choices in inpatient therapy did all of us who work in health care delivery a great disservice. The maligning by politicians and pundits in the media of potential therapies and protection protocols by one organization or another made care at the bedside incredibly confusing and ultimately changeable as each day progressed. I was extraordinarily pleased that within the VHA, the care delivery leadership teams debated these issues and moved forward together as a cohesive collegial team throughout the many months of evolving understanding of this new virus and its response to possible therapies.

There are few examples in history of emerging new disease therapies having this level of public scrutiny. Medical advances and clearly defined protocols for new disease treatments mature slowly as experience and ongoing research move medical care delivery protocols forward toward safe and effective outcomes. The public comment regarding emerging therapies often reflected the fear many elected leaders were experiencing. Their public comments were often a disservice to those who were working continuously to deliver effective and evidence-based care. This often politically charged debate profoundly confused the public, thus disrupting patient and provider relationships as choices in therapy became political talking points rather than risk benefit-defined choices delivered purely within the context of patient care decisions. Some state governors even threatened criminal prosecution of providers delivering newly available or newly considered medications for COVID-19 patients that were publicly promoted by a elected leader. I can think of no other disease since smallpox variolation in Boston in the 1720s that elicited as much public controversy over choices in pharmaceutical and medical care than COVID-19.

I absolutely believe that patients have the right to receive and should expect a safe environment when they enter a health care facility. Protection from disease should include assurance that your health care provider team has taken all actions to protect you from infection, even by the team that will provide your actual care. If that includes immunization, then every health care worker who does not show evidence of effective natural immunity should be immunized to reduce risk in patients they care for.

I am aware that this may be a controversial position. Let me relate a story of an actual Veteran patient admitted for complex cancer surgery at a major Midwest (non-VHA) university hospital. He survived his cancer surgery but developed COVID-19 from an unimmunized but asymptomatic COVID-19 positive health care worker. He was discharged home to his family early in the post-operative period because he was COVID-19 positive. He was discharged into the care of his wife who was in active therapy for advanced cancer. She then developed COVID-19 while diligently and lovingly caring for her husband. They have both survived, but the toll on each was significant and resulted in the subsequent admission of the Veteran to a VAMC COVID-19 unit for continued care. There are those who would debate the outcomes if the care team was immunized. I am convinced that we must provide every possible protection for our patients that is possible.

CHAPTER TWENTY-ONE

Vaccine and Hope

THE VHA, AS PART of its massive research organization, was an active and significant participant in the development of each vaccine that would eventually be licensed by the Food and Drug Administration (FDA) under what is termed an "emergency use authorization" (EUA). The first EUA came on Dec 11, 2020, with the Pfizer vaccine. This was a new type of vaccine using what is called messenger RNA to trigger the patient's immune response. We had anxiously awaited the vaccine's arrival as our hope was that it would reduce the risk of severe disease in those patients at high risk of serious disease or death. It was also a chance to protect our workforce. By December 11th of 2020, we had lost nearly seventy-five hundred Veterans who had died from infection with the COVID-19 virus. Our hospitals were filled with thousands of COVID-19-infected patients, and our staff was at near breaking point from exhaustion. The EUA of the Pfizer vaccine brought hope that there was relief coming soon, hope that the operational pace would decline, hope that Americans could live their lives normally again, and hope that there might be an end to what had now reached a year of pandemic response.

The first dose of vaccine delivered to the VHA was administered to a ninety-six-year-old WWII Veteran at the Bedford, Massachusetts, VA Medical Center on December 14, 2020. We had been planning for the vaccine and distribution for months by ensuring the availability of what is termed "ultra-cold" freezers that would protect the stability of the vaccine until it was needed. We had a number of these ultra-cold freezers because they were used in our medical research. We were fortunate, however, that Deb Kramer's logistics and acquisition team had secured enough additional freezers early enough in the process to provide vaccine storage to thirty-seven sites around the nation.

When the first doses arrived on our campus, employees were waiting outside in anticipation of the vaccine arrival and began to run after the truck as it approached the loading dock. This scene of employees waiting outside for the arrival of the truck carrying the vaccine and then cheering as it came into view was repeated at virtually every medical center across the VHA as the vaccine packages arrived. There was laughter and singing and thank you' s extended to the truck drivers who delivered these packages of the vaccine. Within a few hours, we began offering the vaccine to our most high-risk employees in the ERs and ICUs. This was followed by vaccinating our at-risk Veterans and then eventually their spouses and caregivers as supplies of the vaccine increased. Employees lined up by the hundreds at each VA facility, and the processes went smoothly across the VHA enterprise. Steve Lieberman was the silent hero in all of this work as he negotiated the distribution of the vaccine to VHA in the CDC, FDA, and HHS daily vaccine work group meetings. Steve had earned the trust of the ASPR team and HHS by this time, and all understood the value of a healthy

VHA workforce to the national pandemic response. The sheer volume of at-risk Veterans across the nation was also clear to all.

A week later, on the 18th of December, the Moderna vaccine was licensed under the same EUA FDA approval model. The advantage of the Moderna product was that it could be stored in a normal freezer and did not require the special refrigeration units the Pfizer product required. We distributed this product, therefore, more broadly and to more remote locations. The arrival of these vaccines was met with the same enthusiasm by employees that we had seen during the first week. The presence of two different vaccines with different dilution requirements and storage requirements created a significant concern for reliable processes across the mammoth delivery system with 175 hospitals, 132 extended-care facilities, and more than 1200 ambulatory care sites. The pharmacy team under the direction of VHA pharmacy chief Mike Valentino led the storage, preparation, and delivery of the vaccine flawlessly.

I received my first dose of vaccine on the 18th of December at the Washington, DC, VA medical center. I was eligible because I received my personal health care from that medical center and was in the high-risk age group. The vaccine caused a few minor side effects, including some uncomfortable chest pain the first night, but within twenty-four hours, I felt fine and remained at work. It is difficult to describe the relief that I experienced with the vaccination. It was as if a yearlong nightmare had the potential of coming to an end. I couldn't describe this well until I began personally delivering vaccinations to fellow employees and others at central office. The response was the same on all my trips around the country.

The VHA had developed profoundly efficient processes for delivery and the administration of the vaccine and had significant delivery capacity beyond Veterans, their caregivers, and our VA employees. We, therefore, chose to support local communities that were struggling with staffing or operating vaccine delivery sites for their communities. We accepted a mission from HHS to support the Bronx borough in New York City, a forty-two square mile area. The vaccination administration site we were assigned to was an aged brick building serving as an armory of the New York National Guard. I asked to participate in assisting the vaccine delivery at this site in order to understand what the providers were actually doing and how it was impacting patients. This is primarily a Spanish-speaking area of the Bronx, and I was assigned, therefore, a Spanish-speaking interpreter. As I gave the vaccine injections, almost every recipient had a story that related to how the pandemic had affected them personally or their families. Many more than I expected had lost a loved one to the virus, and many wept for their loss as they received their vaccine and related their stories. They each lamented that their deceased loved one had died before the vaccine was available. After a few had related their stories, my interpreter and I were wiping away our own tears. We talked at the end of my time giving vaccines, and she related her own loss during the pandemic and that she had volunteered for this clinic because she wanted to be close to everyone who had hope for the future. For me, this was a connection point— all the isolation of the pandemic, losses sustained alone, and now we were seeing our own pain reflected in others, our hope reflected in others. That's what the vaccine brought all of us, hope; not for a cure but that the fear of dying from this awful disease could possibly be reduced.

I found the same stories in every vaccine clinic that I worked. It impressed me that when I worked the vaccination clinic inside

VA central office, we vaccinated many employees who had not been into the workplace for nearly a year. They all had similar stories of loss in their families and the impression that their time at home was isolating them from their fellow employees and the emotional support structure their fellow employees represented. I had the opportunity to vaccinate, among others, VA attorneys from the Office of General Counsel and employees of the Veterans Benefit Administration. The stories were the same, long periods of loneliness, loss, and profound hope for the future.

There has been a lot written about what percentage of various demographic groups received the vaccine. My experience was that the vaccine was accepted most by those who had experienced the most death and disability from the disease. The ER, ICU, and anesthesia providers and staff received the vaccine in very high rates. Because we protected very well the elderly Veteran population confined to the VHA extended-care facilities, the staff there accepted the vaccine at a lower rate unless their families had experienced death or severe disease. The final analysis revealed acceptance of the vaccine by VHA's more than 363,000 employees exceeded 95 percent. During my tenure that ended in July 2021, we did not make vaccination mandatory. I made this decision because of the EUA licensing and the broad voluntary acceptance of the vaccine by the workforce.

It is notable that vaccination rates of all types are lower in communities of color than in predominantly white communities. One reason for vaccine hesitancy in communities of color in the southeast geographic areas of the United States is a remnant of the Tuskegee syphilis study conducted from 1932 to 1972 by the United States government. [46] This study of 400 syphilis-infected Black males who resided in Macon County,

Alabama, denied these patients effective therapy for their disease. Effective therapy was approved in 1947 with the release of penicillin. Penicillin cured the disease of syphilis. Despite that approval, these patients were denied therapy, resulting in more than 128 deaths, forty spouses were infected, and at least nineteen children were born with congenital syphilis. The ultimate release of information regarding this study has tarnished, for good reason, the willingness of communities of color across the southeast portions of the US to accept the US government's information on vaccines now, even fifty years later.

There is one exception to this, and that is among Veterans treated in VHA medical centers. Veterans of color received the COVID-19 vaccination across the nation at higher rates than white Veterans. [47] The highest rate of acceptance of any Veteran demographic subtype was among Black Veterans, followed by Hispanic Veterans and then white Veterans. This was not an anomaly. In many areas of the country, there are health care "deserts," where almost all providers have abandoned a geographic region. In many of these communities, the only remaining provider is the VHA. Early in the summer of 2020, well before the release of the vaccine, the VHA began discussing possible vaccine acceptance with these communities and engaged trusted community influencers over those decisions. The VHA embarked upon significant communication with both patients and community leaders, including faith communities, to provide robust and transparent information about the possible vaccines that might become available. We acknowledged to each of these groups in advance of the EUA the lack of trust the federal government had with these communities. We are gratified that the communities of color inside the Veteran population erased many anticipated disparities. We need to recognize, however, that the same effort needs to be given to rural white male Veterans who have now emerged as those with the lowest vaccination rates. [48]

Erasing disparity in these communities is always a reflection of trust. That trust is earned by a long-term commitment to the community. I have previously written about erasing increased death rates from prostate cancer in Black male Veterans enrolled in VA health care. That effort reflects the trust of those Veterans to receive needed care in the VHA system without financial disincentive. The erasure of financial disincentives to care is a primary cause of the VHA's success and a model that the rest of American health care needs to consider. Each year in the United States, a substantial percentage of provider-prescribed medications are not actually obtained by patients (outside the VHA).[49] These patients are often faced with the economic reality of paying for their medication vs. paying for food or even ensuring stable housing. Food and housing insecurity will become ever-increasing challenges as inflation escalates the cost of those items to those without access to the VHA model of health care. In those Americans with high deductible employer-provided health insurance, the out-of-pocket cost of medications is often paid for by the patient on a high interest credit card or simply the drug prescribed is not obtained. That choice does not have to be made in Veterans enrolled in VHA health care because of minimal or even zero out-of-pocket expense for these medications. One of the hidden barriers to communities of color in access to effective care is the unfathomable decision of needing to choose food and housing over medications prescribed to stabilize acute or chronic health care challenges. The recent emergence of high levels of inflation makes these decisions much more common as increased numbers of Americans face an inability to garner enough financial resources to cover each of these expenses.

CHAPTER TWENTY-TWO

Fear

I HAVE WRITTEN ABOUT THE importance of hope, especially as it pertains to the availability of the COVID-19 vaccine. In this next section, we will focus our attention now on the role of fear in the dynamics of individual and team functionality. There is, in the face of fear, the real risk of becoming individually frozen in place. All of us who have been trained in the military wonder how we will react when we, for the first time, come under enemy fire. Most of us do well, and that is a testament to effective military training. Some, however, become frozen in place for fear of their lives and their wellbeing.

While deployed to Afghanistan, the United States military suffered a helicopter crash with significant loss of coalition service member lives. Unfortunately, due to the crash, all of the victims' bodies were dismembered. The recovery team working at the mountainous crash site was defended by a robust infantry team who protected the perimeter so the work to recover the bodies could continue. The work, however, remained remote, disheartening, and very dangerous. The leader of the personnel recovery team asked for behavioral health support on location of the crash site as the recovery was going to take a number of days, and the soldiers assigned to the recovery operation had never seen or handled dismembered bodies. I agreed to send a behavioral health provider and support technician to the crash site and committed that both would remain until the crash site was cleared. I asked the commander of the behavioral health unit under my command to assign both a provider and technician, and we would fly them to the crash site in a medevac helicopter. An hour later, I was called to the behavioral health clinic to find the chosen provider crouching in a corner, weeping and shaking. This was her first deployment, and she had never anticipated the experience of leaving her clinic to care for those in need. She had never even considered that patients wouldn't come to her in the confines of our compound.

As I considered the options, it was clear that we needed another provider who would inspire confidence from an experienced but demoralized group of war fighters and a team of inexperienced recovery experts who were surrounded by the body parts of their friends and colleagues.

The provider that we removed from the mission never emotionally recovered, and we, unfortunately, removed the provider from the combat theater upon the advice of her commander, another behavioral health provider. The point I am trying to make here is not about the inability of this soldier to perform her mission, which I considered critical for the combat force on the ground at the crash site and for the recovery team. For each of them, the horror of these events and the human toll is real. But the faster we could decompress the stress on them, the more likely they could face future challenges effectively. I introduce these events in order to discuss the impact of fear, fear that overwhelms anything you may have anticipated in your life, and fear that paralyzes you and makes you wonder if you can even maintain your bowel and bladder control. It is my hope that none of you will ever experience that level of fear. Unfortunately, my deployment order led the soldier described over that emotional cliff.

As the pandemic accelerated in January and February 2020, there was little known about the penetrance of the disease in the American population. In addition, of those American's infected with the virus, how sick would they be? How many would need hospitalization, and how many would eventually die? As discussed previously, we also knew little about how many of our own employees we would lose to infection and death. Thus, our ability to sustain our expanded operational posture was in question. Privately, the McKinsey team shared worst-case data from several countries, including Italy, that suggested that without significant proactive actions during the first few months of the medical response to COVID-19, we would become completely overwhelmed and unable to sustain our ability to support the nation. I thought that these must be the same data points the governor of New York was looking at as he called for massive amounts of help.

As the sheer magnitude of this untenable position washed over me, I immediately thought back to that behavioral health provider in Afghanistan and the prospect of becoming frozen by fear. I asked the McKinsey team to consider all possibilities to include a relook of the initial cruise line data from quarantined cruise ship passengers. That data showed a lower actual penetrance of infection by the virus than expected on most ships, and the cruise ship passenger populations were similarly age-matched to Veterans with the cruise ship passengers being substantially older than the rest of the American population. As the team took on this relook of possible scenarios, I transparently discussed with the VHA leadership team the following simple concept that I believe is the key to responding to this type of overwhelming fear. If I am going to fall off a cliff, it doesn't really matter if it's a high cliff or low cliff. What really matters is whether I believe that I have any control over the eventual outcome when I finish falling.

As McKinsey briefed me on the amended data that included the rate of infection and death on quarantine cruise ships, I decided to present that data to the entire VHA management team. I believed that what the McKinsey team had prepared showed that our future was quite possibly in our own control and that actions we could take as a leadership team would have a positive outcome and substantially improve the chance of our eventual success.

One of my mentors discussed with me recently that she can always tell she is in the presence of a battle-hardened military leader when a crisis occurs. She related that there is a calmness around those leaders while everyone else on the team is over-whelmed. True "superpower," she says, is when that calm emanating from the leader can overtake an entire team who can then control their own future in facing a crisis. She believes that I, and the other combat-hardened Veterans in positions of leadership at the VA, provided that calm, that then enabled each VHA leader at every level to take control and ultimately define the organization's future. The presence of a common goal, of saving every life we could, unified the organization's focus at unprecedented levels.

There is significant historical literature about the actions of the British government during WWII as the Nazis began bombarding London and the fear that the government leaders anticipated would overtake the British civilian population. As the bombing began, in fact, there was some of the civilian population immobilized by fear. But, for most of the citizens of London, they survived the bombing, and they responded amazingly well in heroic efforts to support their fellow citizens. The population operated well beyond the predictions of the British government and functioned quite effectively in the face of unbelievable deprivation and suffering. Some part of this response reflected the unwavering leadership and communication skills of the then serving British Prime Minister Winston Churchill. [50]

It was my impression as the leader of the VHA that all of us as leaders must demonstrate the ability to manage our own fear. It is not necessary to deny the existence of fear; in fact, there is evidence that naming the fear can help to address it. But a leader must effectively manage its presence in order to remain in control of one's own future. Only then can a leader manage the future response of the organization that they lead.

When the McKinsey team presented the predictions for the future using amended population data, the VHA leaders responded exactly as I had hoped. They immediately recognized and then developed sequential contingency plans that anticipated various levels of disease penetrance, hospitalization rates, and death. They also developed staged staffing plans for various levels of the workforce unable to work due to infection or quarantine. These contingency plans allowed each of them to manage their own organizational futures. They were able to adjust and transform with an agility that was quite remarkable. Never were they overwhelmed. Even when it seemed they would go over the cliff in a geographic region, they showed the creativity and ingenuity to develop an additional staffing or operating model to expand just a little further than they thought that they could reach the previous day. What they demonstrated, more than anything else, was the ability to have hope and overcome fear. That hope was strengthened by the confidence that their previous success was a foundation to build upon and their confidence that they were not alone in any of these decisions. If they faltered, the rest of the VHA would support them as quickly as possible.

I have thought a lot about that soldier in Afghanistan and how poorly we prepared her for what she might experience. How alone she felt in those moments after she was informed of her mission. There were several ways I could have handled the situation more effectively as her commander. Thankfully, that experience prepared me to face my own fear in the early stages of the pandemic.

CHAPTER TWENTY-THREE

Partisanship — Always Directed to the Benefit of the American Veteran

I HAVE ALWAYS CONSIDERED MYSELF non-political and, like a lot of Americans, I believe that politics is an ugly business. It is my hope that whatever partisanship I demonstrated in my actions was directed solely to improve the wellbeing and health of America's Veterans and uniformed service members. I am disinclined to take political positions or align to a political party as I am convinced that, at various times over the history of the United States, party loyalty has prevented or obstructed good decision-making for the benefit of the nation and its citizens. I am reminded of Ronald Reagan's farewell address to the nation delivered on January 11, 1989 and referenced in a brief essay by Charles Kesler in the Winter 2021/22 issue of the *Clairmont Review of Books*. Reagan said the following in his farewell address, "Those of us who are over thirty-five years of age (born before 1954) grew up in a different America. We were taught, very directly, what it means to be an American. And we absorbed, almost in the air, a love of country and an appreciation of its institutions." [51]

I have always loved this country, and my service to the nation in uniform continued an unbroken family history of service that dates back to the American Revolution. I find myself, therefore, disconnected from those who are ambivalent about America or who believe that America has moved past its Declaration of Independence or its Constitution. I find much of the rhetoric from today's politicians and the media during this incredibly divisive time in our American journey as anti-American or using the words of Kesler, even "post-American."

I think of myself as a traditional American patriot and cannot renege upon the oath of service that I pledged when I raised my right hand and placed my left hand on our family Bible and stated the following:

> I, Richard Stone, do solemnly swear that I will support and defend the Constitution of the United States against all enemies, foreign and domestic; that I will bear true faith and allegiance to the same; that I take this obligation freely, without any mental reservation or purpose of evasion; and that I will well and faithfully discharge the duties of the office on which I am about to enter, so help me God.

This is the oath I took as a uniformed Army officer. I repeated these words with every uniformed promotion. It is the same oath that I took as a civilian senior executive serving at the VHA.

This oath is unique in the world today. There are 193 nations in the world. America is the only one, where a service member or a civil servant pledges their entire being, including the possibility of giving up their own life, to the idea that is their nation; not a political party, not to an individual leader, but pledging their lives to an idea that is unique in human history. For the vast majority of the 57 million Americans who have now served in the uniform of this country since 1776, there exists an unbreakable bond to this idea of America itself.

This very personal preamble leads me to describe the civil unrest that overtook Washington, DC, from the 28th of May to June 23rd of 2020, following the murder of George Floyd in Minneapolis on May 25th. The Washington, DC, VHA central office is located at 810 Vermont Avenue and housed in a hundred-year-old stone building owned by the General Services Administration but branded as the Department of Veterans Affairs. The building sits on the edge of Lafayette Square, a seven-acre park directly north from the White House, separated by Pennsylvania Avenue from the White House grounds. The park is named for Marquis de Lafayette, a French aristocrat and hero of the American Revolutionary War. In the park are statues of European Revolutionary War heroes, and at its center is a statue of General and President Andrew Jackson. North of the park is H Street, and the VA central office's south edifice faces H Street. Vermont Ave extends diagonally from the northeast corner of Lafayette Square, and it was this location, in front of our primary building entrance, that was converted into a police and National Guard staging area for the law enforcement response to the demonstrations and violence that occurred in the days following the May 25th murder.

Destruction was indiscriminate in the blocks and the parks around this area, and the Veterans Affairs building was defaced. The blast-resistant first floor windows were shattered and broken, but the building remained secure. The outside stone was spray painted with profane references to Veterans, the police, and the Trump administration. Next door to our building along H Street to the west is the St. John's Episcopal Church, which has served since 1816 as a place of worship for multiple presidents. Kneeling pads with the names of each president are monogramed in the material covering the kneeling pad that sits upon the floor at the location that each American president knelt, prayed, and worshiped. Each week of the pandemic, I had walked to St. John's church and, when the building interior was accessible, knelt and prayed for the wisdom to save as many lives as we could and for my decisions to reflect both wisdom and compassion. In that building, I was surrounded by the echoes of the prayers of many of the nation's greatest patriots. It was a place of peace. On May 31st of 2020 at 10:30 pm, an arsonist firebombed the basement of the church.

I found myself viewing this bombing as an intensely personal attack. An attack meant to destroy a location of solace and worship that had served this nation's most senior leaders for more than two hundred years, a place that I had personally found provided incredible solace and calm. I always felt anchored when I left the church even after a few minutes of quiet solitude and prayer. I often reflected during these times on the last pew in the right rear of the church. Inscribed with the name of Abraham Lincoln, who, it is said, always arrived late for service and in an effort not to disturb others would sit in the last pew on the right. It is rumored that he often succumbed to sleep during the minister's homily.

I was working with my entire team at the VHA headquarters through the worst pandemic in one hundred years. I had found a place to seek solace and a personal connection to my own faith and my love of my country. I, as a leader, could not understand, nor could I connect with the expressed tolerance or even encouragement by elected political officials for organized

SAVE EVERY LIFE YOU CAN

acts of lawlessness around the country. My emotion was based upon fatigue, emotional exhaustion, and, I believe, primarily upon the ongoing deaths of VHA employees from COVID-19 and an inability to reconcile and grieve for those losses. These were government servants whose deaths I had internalized during this time as we continued service to the nation and its heroes that we loved. My own separation from this sacred place of worship following the bombing and ensuing fire became an intensely personal connection to the bombing from which I have still not recovered. The conversion of the broken stained glass and decorative windows at St John's to social justice murals painted over plywood was a constant reminder of the wanton destruction caused by this violence.

This loss was intensely personal.

I will always support and defend the right of Americans to express their views in civil protest. In addition, I support the right to have each of our voices heard while expressing grief, despair, and absolutely rejecting the violence that resulted in the murder of George Floyd. But what I experienced every day around the nation's capital was simply deliberate and wide-spread destruction. On the blocks upon which I worked (and it seemed in multiple other cities across America), I witnessed city, state, and even federal leaders who struggled with their ability to frame these events in a coherent manner. It seemed that the country had lost its way, and there were almost no voices of leaders at any level to foster a climate of reconciliation of these events.

I find that my disconnection from many in this discussion divides along the lines of protest that leads to political change conducted within our election process and those who I believe have moved past America and discarded the fundamental concept that America always was and still remains an exceptional place. I will never waver from my belief in American exceptionalism. This was cemented by many events in my life. Let me enumerate but one. I once stood in Kabul, Afghanistan, on the soccer field where women accused of adultery had been buried up to their necks and then, in the presence of thousands of Afghan citizens who filled the seats of the surrounding stadium, were stoned to death under Taliban rule. I was appalled and sickened at the inhumanity that had occurred and was tolerated. I was incredibly proud that I stood on that soccer field wearing the uniform of the nation that led the coalition that freed women from that intolerable oppression.

Paraphrasing Lincoln's 1862 message to Congress, "America is . . . the last best hope for earth." This belief in the concept of American exceptionalism does not in any way suggest that America is perfect or without problems that must be remedied. But, as I look around the world, there is little that suggests to me anything good will come from rejecting or discarding the idea of, and belief in, American exceptionalism.

The events I have described in the midst of the pandemic response of massive civil unrest and indiscriminate destruction in our cities while the VHA and the nation continued our engagement in the largest public health challenge of the last one hundred years was a low point for me and, I think, many of us on the VHA team. Even now, I remain saddened by the behavior of elected leaders who, it seems, are unable to defend what is good about this nation or even their own communities. This imbalance must be resolved as the country, at some point defines a path forward. Without this type of reconciliation and healing, the possibility of optimism and hope for the future will be very difficult.

CHAPTER TWENTY-FOUR

The Death of My Dad

I LEFT VHA ON JULY 16, 2021, after the Biden administration decided that I would not be selected as their nominee for the Senate-confirmed position of under secretary for health for VHA. I had been selected by a search committee made up of Veteran Service Organizations, former under secretaries, and noteworthy healthcare leadership, and my name was forwarded to the White House. Unfortunately, the White House ultimately decided to go in a different direction. I had been leading the VHA as the acting under secretary or executive in charge for three full years, the longest job interview in history. It was tough to accept that I would not lead the VHA into the future. My relationship with the new Secretary of the VA Denis McDonough, who had been confirmed in February 2021, was excellent. He and I had developed what I believed was an open and productive dialogue on our challenges and the way forward. He expressed to me that he was sincerely saddened that I had not been selected. I remain respectful of the decision and decided it was time to step away from nearly thirty years of uniformed and civilian government service. I announced that I would leave the VHA on July 16, 2021.

I decided that after leaving the VHA, I would take a few months to rest before accepting another challenge. Leaving the VHA team was more emotional than I can describe, and the weeks that went by after the announcement of my non-selection as the nominee for USH was filled with emotional goodbyes. For the most part, these occurred in my office and some (for remote individuals) via video conferences. I described this to one of my mentors as like attending my own wake.

There is an important lesson in all of this for leaders preparing to depart their organizations. First, recognize that not being selected for a job is not a reflection on your ultimate talents or skills. This recommendation is difficult to execute successfully, especially when you are emotionally attached to your hoped-for job. There are so many dynamics to these very high-level jobs and thus so many stakeholders that must be satisfied. For the VHA under secretary for health position, even United States senators may have virtual veto power over a nominee because of some perceived misstep in dealing with them. The message here is, don't take it personally. The other message is sometimes doing what is right has tough consequences for your professional longevity.

Most important is understanding how you behave as a leader as you reach the end of your tenure can either destabilize or stabilize an organization. I am a Veteran receiving my health care from the VHA. I need this organization to remain strong and provide reliable excellence in all its processes, and that requires a stable senior leadership team to provide continuity and carry the progress that we made during my tenure into the future.

Finally, I have always operated under the concept that God puts us wherever we are supposed to be. Get over it. The plan for the future will reveal itself soon enough.

I departed VHA after shedding lots of tears and decided that for the first time since September 11, 2001, my wife Jenni and I would relax and spend a number of months doing nothing at our home in southwest Florida. Eleven days later, on July 27, my 102-year-old dad developed COVID-19 while confined to a memory care unit in Sarasota, Florida.

As I related previously, my dad came into our lives when I was just turning twelve years old. He was everything in a father that I never had. He was loving and engaged in everything in our lives. He was a trained and college-educated musician with an interest in classical music composition and performance piano. When he couldn't make a living at what he loved, he went back to school and was admitted to medical school, where he became an extraordinary physician and teacher of developing physicians. He completely accepted my older brother and me when he married my mom, and we became a family, the cohesiveness of which I had never experienced before he entered our lives.

Many years later, in late 2002, my mom died very suddenly in the months before I deployed to Afghanistan. A few years later, Dad met Judy and experienced a wonderful late-in-life love affair, and they were married, their love persisting even after Dad developed some cognitive decline. His new wife developed some complex immunosuppression, and they found themselves at the beginning of the COVID-19 pandemic with Dad living in a memory care facility and Judy remaining in their home in Sarasota. Dad had a wonderful type of cognitive decline (if there can be such a thing) in that he remembered everything that happened years ago but could not remember if he ate breakfast. Everything in life was a surprise, and he was always delighted to see us visit. He discussed at length events in the distant past, but events earlier in the current day just didn't imprint into his memory. Judy, his wife, was wonderful about visits and was able to take him out of the facility for dinner and outings until COVID-19 came to the Sarasota community. Suddenly, we were all separated and unable to continue our visits with each other.

Dad declined immediately as so many of those confined and experiencing isolation did. The removal of communal dining, group activities, and the presence of masks added to the isolation and decline. He had severe hearing loss, and the assisted living facility was unable to help us maintain possession of multiple sets of eventually lost hearing aids. We spent thousands of dollars on hearing aids that were lost in no more than a month or so. Phone calls with Dad became more and more difficult, and the commercial facility was unable to support other technology-enabled visits. We were able to obtain a headphone-hearing assistance device with a remote microphone that worked remarkably well but required our physical presence to set it up and operate.

During a COVID-19 lull in the Sarasota community in early July, we were able to visit Dad and got the opportunity to be physically present in his room after showing the facility our vaccination cards. We hooked up his hearing device, and he and I watched the news together on the television in his room while I placed the receiver microphone next to the television speaker. Dad went from head down in the recliner to sitting up, wide awake, and conversant. He asked me to define the word "woke." After I explained my understanding of being woke, he asked the same question again. I changed my answer slightly, and then Dad smiled and said the following, "Either way you answer, it doesn't make much sense to me." He then asked me why a cyberattack would focus on hospitals. As I answered him, I decided his cognitive loss was as much just hearing loss-related, and his cognition was better than we had been informed over the many months that we couldn't visit him. That was the last of our visits before he was infected with COVID-19 in spite of his own vaccination.

We received a call on July 27th, eleven days after I left VHA, and were informed that Dad was COVID-19 positive. His doctor who knew him for years was unfortunately not privileged to provide care at the memory care unit he was confined to. In addition, there was no ability for the single physician provider covering the entire memory unit to provide the medical care Dad required, and so Dad was transferred to the largest hospital in Sarasota.

The massive Sarasota-based hospital Dad was transferred into is an 839-bed county government public medical center advertising itself as a full-service health system. After some discussion with both security and nursing at the hospital, my wife Jenni and I were able to visit him. We found him on a COVID-19-positive unit with what appeared to be a supportive staff. Because of COVID-19, our visitation was limited, and we were able to visit only because the care team viewed him to be pre-terminal.

I admit that what follows is memories clouded by the emotion of loss of a loved one.

When we entered his room, we found Dad with thick secretions in his upper respiratory system, precluding swallowing and interfering with his effective breathing. We also found him without any suction unit in the room to remove the obvious secretions. We discussed this with the nursing staff, and they informed us that Dad had been evaluated by the "swallowing experts," and their testing revealed that he could not swallow, and therefore he was not being fed or given oral fluids. My wife (a certified registered nurse anesthetist) and I obtained a suction unit from his nurse, and we actually suctioned his secretions. He was immediately able to swallow without significant difficulty. Despite this, the "cannot swallow" tag remained, and Dad slowly succumbed over a period of days to a lack of calorie intake and fluid depletion. He died on the 19th of August, experiencing a difficult and labored death. I relate all of this because in my forty years of healthcare, I have witnessed difficult and sometimes painful deaths, and my Dad's was one of the most difficult, worsened by bedside care delivered at a standard well below what I saw and expected every day in the VHA that I led.

Conversations during this time with nursing leadership at the commercial hospital informed us, "You know our nurses are involuntarily assigned to the COVID-19 unit." Discussions with the attending physician reflected a need for him to negotiate attempts at feeding and oral fluid intake with the staff. We attempted during this time to bring in a private duty nurse to enhance his care. This proved to be impossible because of COVID-19 restrictions.

My point in this painful recollection of these events is that I found the care so very culturally different from what I knew and expected of the staff of the VHA, and I was heartbroken. The failure of the leadership team of these care units was reflected in their leaders. There was a chance for each of them to inspire confidence that was just not grasped.

I recognize that not many of us have the chance to have our parent as part of our lives for three months short of 103 years, and we are incredibly grateful for his longevity. That said, the brutal realization that his death could have been different will forever be in my memory. The loneliness of his suffering and the inability to advocate for a patient who was too sick to speak, all this returns me to the previous discussion on the loneliness of COVID-19 deaths and should remind each of us that every patient is someone's mom, dad, brother or sister, daughter or son, friend, neighbor, or colleague, and every life is precious.

I had the impression, maybe completely unfairly, that this nursing staff was just exhausted from the never-ending flow of COVID-19 patients. I also believed that their leaders had failed to deliver the leadership skill to allow their frontline caregivers to feel in control of their future.

After Dad's death, I informed my wife that under no circumstances should I become ill should I be taken to a hospital that was not run by the VHA. I wanted to be in a place that respected who I was as a Veteran and as a person. It was, in the end, an emotional response that had little value except to allay my profound sense of loss.

When death comes to a Veteran in a VHA facility, the Veteran is covered with an American flag, and the staff lines the hallways for a final salute as the body is moved to the morgue. Other Veterans and patients, if physically able, participate in the salute as the flag-draped Veteran is moved slowly down the hallways on a wheeled transport bed. This final salute is eerily the same as what I participated in while deployed to Afghanistan and one of the many things that makes VHA facilities just culturally different from what I experienced at the massive commercial hospital that cared for Dad.

One of my great regrets is that Dad never enrolled in VHA health care and that I was convinced his Sarasota concierge doctor could ensure the quality of his care. I was right until he needed highly competent and well-led nursing care, and then it just wasn't available.

I know that my basic premise that "God puts you wherever you're supposed to be" was why I was called upon to leave the VHA and thus had time to support Dad and Judy in his final days. Judy was never able to see him once he had COVID-19, and her heart broke for the inability to grieve at his bedside and say goodbye. It reminds me of why I think the American health care system needs massive transformation in order to ensure care is available that acknowledges the patient's humanity. The provision of that care must integrate the provision of the patient's acute needs with their long-term caregivers. It is only by fully integrating with those caregivers that a care delivery team can fully understand the patient and their family's needs.

American civilian health care is very good at acute transactions of emergent care. The system is much less adept at the treatment of long-term chronic diseases. Stabilization of uncontrolled hypertension or diabetes mellitus works very well in episodes of acute exacerbation, but routine maintenance care is much more fragmented, and the transitions of care between hospital and ambulatory or home-based settings are very difficult. Stabilizing patients and then the sustainment of that stability in patients needing chronic care is almost always a challenge in the non-VHA setting. Communication between care teams is often the single point of failure in care transitions. Massive financial reimbursement incentives promote magnificent facilities like what we experienced at the commercial hospital in Sarasota, but facilities like this fail in a spectacular and very painful fashion when caring for chronic, debilitated patients with complex comorbid conditions. The death of my own father is a poignant example of why the VHA works as a model for all American health care. Profound care integration accompanied by a lifetime commitment to the care of the Veteran patient is what delivers a dramatically different model of care provided by a unique, mission-focused care team.

In surveys of Veterans receiving care at the VHA, nearly 90 percent of Veterans trust the VHA with their care and recommend VHA care to other Veterans.[52] These numbers are refreshed each week on a continuous basis. I am also reminded that every patient is a unique and extraordinary individual.

My dad was blessed with a loving spouse and family at the time of his death. As he was buried at the Sarasota Federal Veterans Cemetery, he was greeted there by the VA National Cemetery Administration staff with the respect and loving kindness that he was denied while hospitalized over the last few days of his life. I will miss him very much.

CHAPTER TWENTY-FIVE

Conclusion

THE HEROES OF THE VHA COVID-19 response are the tens of thousands of patient-facing VHA employees and their support teams who, by all measures, risked their own lives each and every day to provide care to the patients the VHA was fortunate enough to serve. These extraordinary employees' individual and collective bravery and professionalism inspired each of us every single day, and their ingenuity and creative talent overcame immense risk to our success. All of us who participated in the response to this pandemic are hopeful that another hundred years will transpire before the next public health challenge of the magnitude of COVID-19 engages the world. We need to acknowledge today, however, that as of now, we as a nation just aren't ready.

Regardless of the duration of time until the next challenge we experience as a nation, the stability we experience today is our window of opportunity to prepare for that inevitable day when chaos returns. This generation of pandemic-tested health care leaders will soon fade away, and the ability for us to memorialize the extraordinary events and emotions of the pandemic that began in December 2019 is the ultimate purpose of this book. That this document might lend support to that future generation of medical leaders is the ultimate and fervent hope of the author.

That said, there are two more immediate goals for this work. The first is to memorialize the lessons learned in what could have been a more effective response so a future public health and complex health care delivery challenge can be more easily addressed. These lessons are summarized throughout the book as recommendations and suggested policy and operational changes. This must include sincere and transparent debate by the nation's leaders on the expansion of US-based medical and pharmaceutical manufacturing, effective healthcare coordination between federal and non-federal providers, and a permanent NSC-like apparatus to coordinate the government's future response capability.

The second goal of the author is to provide a substantial window into the development, thought processes, and values of a leader who was called upon to use every leadership experience and tool acquired over a lifetime of leadership positions in order to build an effective team and lead it toward success under the most dire of circumstances. It was an extraordinary privilege to lead the men and women of the Veterans Health Administration during these trying times, and while my decisions were not always perfect, the great government servants of the VHA certainly covered for me. I could not be more proud of what this team and each of them accomplished on behalf of our nation's Veterans and the United States of America.

It is my sincere hope that these pages serve to help future leaders "save every life you can!" It is, in the end, the most important thing any of us can do.

THE END

ANNEX A

Lessons Learned and Recommendations

THE PROCESS OF WRITING this book and the many itera-
tions of it that were developed forced me to think deeply about
who I am as a leader and person in an unexpectedly personal
way. In so doing, I attempted to capture the lessons I have
learned throughout my life and document them here for others
to consider in no particular order:

- Lessons in leadership can occur in any venue if you are
  listening.

- Accept the fact that "to err is human."

- A leader can only lead effectively by physically moving
  around his/her areas of responsibility to see and hear
  with their own eyes and ears the challenges their organizations face. There is no substitute for this.

- God gives me the stability of today to prepare for the
  chaos of tomorrow. Use today wisely.

- Crises that challenge a large organization require risk-taking on the part of leaders to steer a path to success. If you wait for every bit of information to ensure your decision is without risk, the crisis will overtake you.

- If a decision is wrong, don't be afraid to transparently change course. Showing your own ego is in check will help the entire organization make rapid decisions in a crisis.

- Employees will follow leaders who are reliable and predictable in their responses to difficult problems.

- Heroism is often very quiet.

- The sustainment of transformational change requires organizational followership for the concept or process being instituted. Transformation must be more than the pet project of a popular leader if it is to survive from one leader to the next.

- Learning from history will prevent you from repeating the mistakes of the past.

- Leaders must always follow the 25-percent rule: Look for the 25 percent of employees who share your vision and empower them to reach success. The vast majority of others will follow. Do not spend an overt amount of time on the naysayers.

- Leaders must ensure that they never face a crisis with one of anything. This will become the single point of failure from which you cannot recover.

- Crisis communication to your workforce must be frequent, honest, and conducted by you, the leader. Ensure your voice is heard directly by every employee using consistent but creative media techniques. Avoid having multiple layers of subordinate leadership interpret what you said.

- The presence of a contrarian helps a leadership team develop a stronger decision. A contrarian is not an obstructionist. Contrarians provide alternative courses of action. Obstructionists resist proposed action or decisions in favor of the status quo. Always view a contrarian as a key partner in future success.

- When faced with debate in the leadership team, solicit input and listen. Always listen. It enhances followership for subsequent decisions made.

- When not selected for a hoped-for job promotion, your actions as a leader will significantly influence the subsequent performance of your organization. Act graciously.

- The fact that you weren't selected for a job is often not a reflection of your own talents and ability. The higher you get the more elements of your environment impact such things.

- Always attempt, even in the face of fear, to be the leader who provides calm in the center of the storm.

There are a myriad of lessons learned for government that can be reviewed in detail in the VHA-developed COVID-19 After Action Report and subsequent annexes. These are publicly available on the VA website. Some of the key recommendations that I want to emphasize here include the following:

1. Strengthen the roll of the HHS ASPR as the key federal government official and coordinator of medical care delivery response in future public health crises.

2. This first recommendation should include the development, implementation, and sustainment of a **care coordination council** composed of federal health care delivery agencies (DOD, VHA, USPHS, NIH, and IHS). This care delivery council should develop the operating processes to enable the rapid acceptance for federal mission assignment of state requests for support.

3. Review and strengthen the enabling legislation in the 2012 Biodefense Act and the 2012 Presidential Executive Order that could enable number one.

4. Congress should mandate the expansion of ESF 8 in order to enhance care coordination and clearly define crisis casualty management command and control.

5. Develop regional public health crisis simulation exercises, conducted under the authority of the ASPR,

that are conducted regularly to ensure there is understanding of those processes that promote future cohesive patient care between federal, tribal, and commercial delivery networks.

6. Develop a crisis health operations interfacility communication system that increases communication between critical care and emergency providers.

7. Acknowledge and correct immediately the lack of US-based medical and pharmaceutical manufacturing and consider it a national security threat.

8. Replicate the model of DOD's "war stopper" medical material supply management inside VHA.

9. Develop (through the ASPR) robust state and tribal-directed training tools to enhance the ability of state and tribal governments to request federal assistance during future medical crises. Ensure federal systems have authority to respond to those requests in a timely manner.

10. Consider a National Security Council type model (currently used to respond to national defense threats) for future federal response to medical threats.

11. Enhance the ability of medical providers to deliver care across state lines and deliver care at the "top of their licenses," especially during crisis response.

12. Reexamine America's emergency care transportation capabilities and response systems across the United States. This should provide special emphasis on rural and disadvantaged communities' ability to receive care.

13. Develop enabling legislation that enhances Medicare and commercial insurance benefit packages to include long-term care for those who can no longer be cared for at home.

14. Enhance professional staffing mandatory guidelines for long-term assisted living, nursing homes, and skilled nursing homes.

15. Incentivize the development of expanded insurance benefit packages that include in home patient care and enhanced coverage of point-of-service testing conducted in the home.

16. Strengthen those laws that allow VHA oversight of State Veteran Homes to include the ability of VHA to assume temporary operational control of failing facilities.

17. Promote the development of geriatric care paraprofessionals to enhance the reach of the professional registered nurse.

18. Reexamine US government acquisition authorities to enhance the ability to acquire crisis response materials when payment in advance is demanded.

19. Direct the VHA to reexamine and develop mitigating systems for the "just in time" material management processes that failed during the COVID-19 pandemic.

20. Expand laws that enable and promote public private partnerships across the VHA .

ANNEX B

Glossary of Abreviations

ASPR – Assistant Secretary for Preparedness and Response (HHS)

API – Active pharmaceutical ingredient

APRN – Advance Practice Registered Nurse

A-10 – An Air Force subsonic attack aircraft

C-17 – A large military transport aircraft often referred to as the "Globemaster"

CARES ACT – Coronavirus Aid, Relief and Economic Security Act

CDC – Centers for Disease Control and Prevention

CEO – Chief Executive Officer

CG – Commanding General

CJTF – Combined Joint Task Force

CMS – Centers for Medicare and Medicaid Services

COL – Colonel

COO – Chief Operating Officer

COVID-19 – The WHO term for the coronavirus infectious disease caused by the SARS-CoV-2 virus

CPR – Cardiopulmonary resuscitation

CRNA – Certified Registered Nurse Anesthetist

DEA – Drug Enforcement Administration

DO – Doctor of Osteopathy

DOD – Department of Defense

DPA – Defense Production Act

Ebola Virus – Cause of Ebola Hemorrhagic Fever

ESF 8 – Emergency Support Function number 8: Public Health and Medical Services Annex

EUA – Emergency Use Authorization

Executive Order 13603 – 2012 National Defense resources preparedness order

FEMA – Federal Emergency Management Agency

FDA – Food and Drug Administration

FIRST – For Inspiration and Recognition of Science and Technology

GAO – Government Accountability Office

HHS – Department of Health and Human Services

HOC – Health Operations Center

HRO – High Reliability Organization

ICU – Intensive Care Unit

IG – Inspector General

IHS – Indian Health Service

MD – Medical Doctor

MISSION ACT – Maintaining Internal Systems and Strengthening Integrated Outside networks

N95 – A personally fitted respiratory protective device (mask)

NCA – National Cemetery Administration

NCO- Non-commissioned officer

NOVAMC – New Orleans VA Medical Center

OEM- Office of Emergency Management

OIT – Office of Information and Technology

OPM – Office of Personnel Management

OR – Operating room

PAPR – Powered air-purifying respirator

PPE – Personal protective equipment

R0 – Pronounced "R naught" and used in epidemiology to signify the reproductive ability of an infection

RN – Registered nurse

RNA – Ribonucleic acid

SAIL – Strategic Analytics for Improvement and Learning

SME – Subject matter expert

Stafford Act – 1988 Robert Stafford Disaster Relief and Emergency Assistance Act.

USH – Under Secretary for Health VHA

USPHS – United States Public Health Service

VA – Department of Veterans Affairs

VBA – Veterans Benefit Administration

VHA – Veterans Health Administration

VISN- Veteran Integrated Service Network

WHO – World Health Organization

Endnotes

1 "Department of Veterans Affairs COVID-19 National Summary", VA Access to Care, accessed June 25, 2022, https://www.accesstocare.va.gov.

2 Barry, The Great Influenza, 4.

3 "Johns Hopkins Coronavirus Resource Center". Accessed June 30, 2022, https://www.coronavirus.jhu.edu.

4 Ibid.

5 "Lecture on Discoveries and Inventions", accessed August 13, 2022, https://abrahamlincolnonline.org.

6 "Department of Veteran Affairs COVID-19 National Summary", VA Access to Care, accessed June 25, 2022, https://www.accesstocare.va.gov.

7 Wang, "2021 Survey of Veteran Enrollees' Health and Use of Health care", 1-32.

8 "Veteran trust in VA health care rises above 90 percent for the first time", VA Office of Public and Intergovernmental Affairs, April 30, 2020, https://va.gov/opa/pressrel.

9 "Stafford Act", FEMA Disaster Authorities, accessed June 20, 2022, https://www.fema.gov/disaster.

10 ibid.

11   "Number of all hospital beds in the U.S. 1975-2019", accessed August 1, 2022, https://statista.com.

12   "COVID-19 Timeline", accessed July 5, 2022, https://www.cdc.gov/museum.

13   "COVID-19 and Italian Healthcare Workers from the Initial Sacrifice to the mRNA Vaccine:...", accessed June 17, 2022, https://www/frontiersin.org/articles.

14   "Coronavirus Disease New Cases and Deaths", New York Times, accessed May 20, 2022, https://nytimes.com.

15   "The effective reproductive number of the Omicron variant of SARS-CoV-2", Accessed June 12, 2022, https://www.ncbi.nlm,nih.gov.

16   "A timeline of USNS Comfort's short and dramatic stay in New York City", Accessed Aug 1, 2020, www.businessinsider.com.

17   Ibid.

18   Jensen, email message to author, June 20, 2022.

19   "How Many Americans Died in WW1 – History on the Net", accessed May 20, 2022, https://historyonthenet.com.

20   "General Omar Bradley and the remaking of the Veterans administration", accessed March, 20 2022, https://www.va.gov.

21   "National Center for Veteran Analysis and Statistics", accessed February 1, 2022, https://www.va.gov/vetdata.

22   "COVID-19 and Italian Healthcare workers from the initial Sacrifice the mRNA Vaccine...", accessed June 17, 2022, https://www/frontiersin.org.

23   Barry, John, *The Great Influenza.*

24   Novak, "Now closed McCormick Place COVID-19 hospital cost taxpayers $15M to staff, run", Chicago Sun Times, November 13, 2020, https://chicago.sun.times.com.

25   "Average Age of U.S. Hospitals is Increasing", accessed February 22, 2022, https://blog.spacemed.com.

26   "FACT SHEET: The American Jobs Plan supports Veterans", The White House Briefing Room posted April 15, 2021, accessed February 22, 2022, https://www.whitehouse.gov/briefing-room/-releases/2021/04/15.

27   "Sanatorium-from the first to the last", accessed February 20 2022, https://tbfacts.org.

28   "The 25-50-25 Principal of Change – John Maxwell", accessed May 20, 2022, https://www.johnmaxwell.com.

29   Talib, The Black Swan, Prologue.

30   "About ASPR", accessed 14 August 2022, https://aspr.hhs.gov.

31   Waxman, "Coronavirus is putting the U.S. Strategic Stockpile to the Test. Here's the Surprising Story Behind the Stash", Time, March 11, 2020.

32   "Veterans Health Administration Hospitals outperform Non-VHA hospitals in Most Healthcare markets", The Dartmouth Institute, December 10, 2018, https://tdi.dartmouth.edu.

33   Danielle, "The Golden Age of House Calls and Home Physicians Returns", August 16, 2017, https://www.md-athome.com.

34   Ibid.

35   "Subjective Cognitive Decline", Alzheimer's Disease and healthy Aging, accessed June 1, 2022, https://www.cdc.gov.

36   "16th Michigan Infantry Regiment – Wikipedia", accessed August 14, 2022, https://en.m.wickipedia.org.

37   Anchor, Briana Vannozzi, "More families file claims over COVID-19 deaths at NJ veterans homes", NJ Spotlight News, May19, 2022.

38   Hinkle, Laura, "The impact of COVID-19 in State Veteran Homes", The Council of State Governments, April 30, 2021, https://web.csg.org.

39   "Long term care Statistics", accessed August 10, 2022, https://www.consumeraffairs.com.

40   Kenen, Joanne, "Sadness and Death: Inside the VA's state nursing home disaster", Politico, August 24, 2021.

41   "CMS Oversight of Nursing Facility Staffing Levels – Office of the OIG", accessed August 1, 2022, https://oig.hhs.gov.

42   Stulick, Amy, "Nursing Homes See Lowest Cost Increase Among Long-Term Care Settings in 2021", skillednursing-news.com, Feb 16, 2022.

43   "How the world ran out of everything". Accessed August 10, 2022, NY Times, https://www.nytimes.com.

44   "What is an Active Pharmaceutical Ingredient (API)?, Global Pharma Tek, December 12, 2020.

45   "Global Spending on Medicines 2026 forecast", accessed August 1 2022, https://www.statisica.com.

46   "Tuskegee Syphilis Study", Wikipedia, accessed July 19, 2022, https://en.m.wikipedia.org

47 Haderlein, Taona, "Racial / Ethnic Variation in Veteran Health Administration COVID-19 Vaccine Uptake", American Journal of Preventive Medicine, August 27, 2021.

48 Ibid.

49 Norton, Amy, "Many patients may never fill new prescriptions", Reuters health, February 17, 2010.

50 "Comparing the psychological response during the COVID-19 pandemic and Blitz", Lancet, August 27, 2020.

51 Kesler, Charles, "Alien Nation", Clairmont Review of Books, Winter 2021/22.

52 "Veteran Trust in VA health care rises above 90 percent for the first time", VA Office of Public and Intergovernmental Affairs, April 30, 2020.

CPSIA information can be obtained
at www.ICGtesting.com
Printed in the USA
BVHW031502190922
647171BV00002B/2

9 781662 853425